JOHN MUIR TRAIL
DATA BOOK

Other titles of interest:

John Muir Trail: The Essential Guide to Hiking America's Most Famous Trail
John Muir Trail: Special Digital-Only Edition for Northbound Hikers

Pacific Crest Trail: Southern California
Pacific Crest Trail: Northern California
Pacific Crest Trail: Oregon & Washington
Pacific Crest Trail Data Book
Day & Section Hikes Pacific Crest Trail: Southern California
Day & Section Hikes Pacific Crest Trail: Northern California
Day & Section Hikes Pacific Crest Trail: Oregon
Day & Section Hikes Pacific Crest Trail: Washington
One Best Hike: Mt. Whitney

JOHN MUIR TRAIL
DATA BOOK

Elizabeth Wenk

 WILDERNESS PRESS . . . *on the trail since 1967*

John Muir Trail Data Book

1st Edition
Copyright © 2014 by Wilderness Press
Front and back cover photos copyright © 2014 by Elizabeth Wenk
Unless otherwise noted, all interior photos by Elizabeth Wenk
Maps: Elizabeth Wenk
Cover design: Scott McGrew
Editor: Amber Kaye Henderson

ISBN: 978-0-89997-770-6; eISBN: 978-0-89997-771-3
Manufactured in the United States of America

Published by: **Wilderness Press**
 c/o Keen Communications
 PO Box 43673
 Birmingham, AL 35243
 800-443-7227; FAX 205-326-1012
 wildernesspress.com

Visit our website for a complete listing of our books and for ordering information.

Distributed by Publishers Group West
Front cover: Ascending the west side of Mt. Whitney
Back cover: Lake near the Bench Lake Ranger Station

CONTENTS

INTRODUCTION

The John Muir Trail (or, more simply, the JMT) is one of the world's premier long-distance hiking trails. A little more than 220 miles in length, it traverses the spine of California's Sierra Nevada, passing through superb mountain scenery. This is a land of 13,000- and 14,000-foot peaks, of soaring granite cliffs, of lakes by the thousands, and of canyons 5,000 feet deep. The trail passes near roads only in Tuolumne Meadows and Devils Postpile, otherwise winding through remote mountain landscape. Part of the beauty of this long-distance walk is that the landscape continually changes as you travel from Happy Isles (in eastern Yosemite Valley) to Whitney Portal (west of the town of Lone Pine, in the Owens Valley). Each day you will find new wonders to captivate your attention—rounded domes in Tuolumne Meadows, volcanic features near Devils Postpile, magical hemlock forests near Silver Pass, dashing cascades along Bear Creek, the glacial landscape of Evolution Basin, the near-vertical peaks of the Palisades, carpets of alpine flowers around Pinchot Pass, spectacular lake basins such as the Rae Lakes, scattered foxtail pines on Bighorn Plateau, and of course the views from the summit of Mt. Whitney, California's tallest peak. The Sierra is an especially lovely area for a multi-week hike, for it is blessed with the mildest, sunniest climate of any major mountain range in the world. Though rain does fall in the summer, it seldom lasts more than an hour or two, and the sun is out and shining most hours of the day. Most likely the greatest challenge you will face is the logistics of resupplying food because the southern 160 miles do not pass a road, and for the final 110 miles you do not even pass close to a food resupply "depot." You are, of course, not the only person to have heard of these attractions and will encounter people daily, but the trail really is a thin line through a vast land; with little effort you can always camp on your own if you leave the trail.

Using This Book

This book is an abbreviated version of *John Muir Trail: The Essential Guide to Hiking America's Most Famous Trail*, also published by Wilderness Press. This title includes only the data sections of its parent book, including tables with junction locations and distances between junctions, a table of campsite locations, topographic maps, and some basic information to help you plan your trip. If you are seeking a trail description, natural history of the region, possible side trips along the trail, or information on how to hike in the Sierra, I recommend that you purchase the thicker volume; if it proves to be too heavy for the trail, you can keep it for your library and carry a copy of this book.

The goal of this guide is to provide you with the data you need to design your own trip, in advance or as you walk. Some people hike only 7 miles a day while others happily cover more than 20. Some hikers complete the entire trail in one go, while others hike a section at a time. This book should cater to everyone, for it provides information on distances along the trail, established camping locations, stretches of trail with steep ascents and descents, and lateral trails that access the JMT. From there, you design the itinerary that best suits you.

The introductory material provides information on three essential topics: how to obtain a wilderness permit, how to get yourself to and from the two endpoints using either public transportation or a private shuttle, and how to arrange food resupplies along the trail. All the phone numbers and Web addresses required for your planning are supplied. Also provided are maps of Yosemite Valley, Tuolumne Meadows, and Lone Pine to orient you at trailheads.

Next are 17 topographic maps, onto which trail junctions and campsites (listed beginning on page 88) have been plotted.

The topographic maps are followed by the trail data. Mimicking the organization of the larger JMT book, the trail information is split into 13 sections, one for each of the river drainages through which the JMT passes. Each section includes a detailed elevation profile of the trail and a table listing major waypoints, including most trail junctions. Each entry includes the elevation, UTM coordinates, distance from the previous point, and cumulative distance from the JMT endpoints, here given as Happy Isles and Whitney Portal. Elevations, with the exception of those benchmarked by the USGS, have been rounded to the closest 10 feet. The UTM coordinates follow the North American datum 1927, as this is the reference system used on most USGS 7.5-minute maps (as well as the popular Tom Harrison maps). GPS devices and mapping software packages use NAD 1983 as a default, but the coordinates can easily convert between the two reference systems.

At the end of the book is a collection of panoramic photos as well as some extra data tables. The photos have been taken from atop passes, and many of the prominent peaks visible are labeled. Following the panoramas is a table listing established, legal campsites. For each campsite, information provided includes the cumulative trail distance, the UTM coordinates (again NAD 1927), a brief description, and whether campfires are permitted. This is followed by tables with emergency numbers for the jurisdictions through which the JMT passes and the locations of wilderness ranger stations in Sequoia and Kings Canyon National Parks, as well as a table with the locations of permanent food-storage lockers (colloquially known as bear boxes). The final table lists basic information on lateral trails feeding into the JMT, which is useful if you plan to section-hike the JMT or if you unexpectedly need to exit the wilderness and need to determine the most efficient way to exit.

And finally, I wish you a wonderful trip along the JMT. Enjoy the superb surroundings as you traipse along a trail that commemorates one of the world's most influential conservationists.

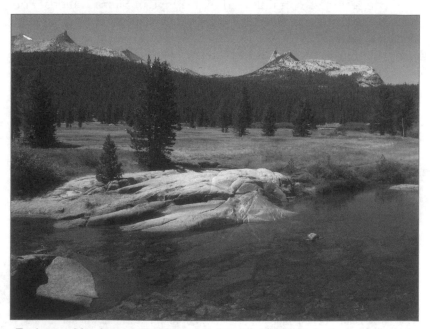

Tuolumne Meadows with Unicorn and Cathedral Peaks in the background

PLANNING YOUR HIKE

Wilderness Permits

All trailheads accessing the JMT require a wilderness permit and have quotas. For all Sierra wilderness areas, permits are issued for the trailhead and date at which you begin your hike. You do not need to obtain a new permit after exiting the wilderness for a food resupply. If you are getting a permit issued by the Inyo or Sierra National Forests and are exiting at Whitney Portal, you are subject to Mt. Whitney Zone exit quotas (25 people per day). A word of warning: Quotas for reserved permits fill very quickly in summer. Reserve your permit as soon as they become available and, if possible, have alternate, weekday start dates as potential backups.

Permit Offices

Yosemite National Park Wilderness Permit Office
nps.gov/yose/planyourvisit/wildpermits.htm
Note: If you begin your walk in Yosemite, you will most likely use one of three permits: Happy Isles to Little Yosemite Valley (if you plan to spend your first night at the Little Yosemite Valley campsite), Happy Isles to Sunrise/Merced Lake (pass-through; if you plan to spend your first night at the Clouds Rest junction or beyond), or Lyell Canyon (if you plan to begin your southbound hike in Tuolumne Meadows).

Inyo National Forest Wilderness Permit Offices
recreation.gov (for reservations)
www.fs.usda.gov/inyo (look under Passes & Permits, then Recreation Passes & Permits for information)
Note: If you are departing from Whitney Portal, you will need a permit for the Mt. Whitney Trail, available only by a lottery held in February.

High Sierra Ranger District (Sierra National Forest)
tinyurl.com/sierrapermit

Sequoia and Kings Canyon National Parks
nps.gov/seki/planyourvisit/wilderness_permits.htm

Permit Reservation Information

Agency	When to Reserve	How to Reserve	Cost	Percent of Permits Available for Reservation	First-Come, First-Serve Permit Availability
Yosemite NP	24 weeks in advance	Phone, mail, fax*	$5 per permit + $5 per person	60%	11 a.m. day before entry
Inyo NF	6 months in advance	Internet	$6 per permit + $5 per person**	60%	11 a.m., day before entry, but can fill in request form at 8 a.m.
Whitney Portal (Inyo NF)	February 1, by lottery	Internet	$15 per person	100%	Only cancellations available
Sierra NF	1 year in advance	Mail	$5 per person	60%	Wilderness station opening, day before entry
Sequoia/Kings Canyon NP	March 1	Mail, fax	$15 per group	75%	1 p.m., day before entry

* You can fax in permits after the office closes at 5 p.m. PST the day before.
Applications received by this method are processed in random order at 8 a.m. the following morning.
** $15 per person if exiting at Whitney Portal

Transportation

Listed on the following page are the main public transport agencies you can use to get to and from the Sierra or between trailheads along the JMT corridor. Public transport options to the Sierra are available from airports in the San Francisco Bay Area and Los Angeles International Airport (LAX), as well as from smaller airports, including Mammoth Lakes, Reno, Merced, Bakersfield, Fresno, and Inyokern. Yosemite Area Regional Transportation System (YARTS) buses deliver you close to trailheads in Yosemite Valley and Tuolumne Meadows. For trailheads in the Mammoth Lakes region, you can take YARTS or Eastern Sierra Transit (EST) buses to the town and then take local EST-run bus services or the Devils Postpile/Reds Meadow bus to the trailheads. To reach trailheads not accessible by public transport, a selection of charter services is available. See the JMT Lateral Trails table on pages 110–112 for additional trail information.

Transit Agency Contact Information

AGENCY	TYPE	WEBSITE	PHONE
Amtrak	Train and bus	amtrak.com	800-AMTRAK-2 (800-268-7222)
Antelope Valley Airport Express	Bus	antelopeexpress.com	800-251-2529
Bay Area Rapid Transit (BART)	Commuter Rail	bart.gov	510-465-2278
Eastern Sierra Transit (EST)	Bus	estransit.com/CMS	760-872-1901 or 800-922-1930
Yosemite Area Regional Transit System (YARTS)	Bus	yarts.com	877-989-2787

Transit Route Information

ROUTE	AGENCY	HOURS	FREQUENCY
SFO or OAK ←→ Richmond	BART	1	Every 20–30 minutes
SFO ←→ Embarcadero (SF Financial Center)	BART	0.5	Every 20–30 minutes
SF Financial Center ←→ Emeryville	Amtrak (bus)	0.5	Timed to meet each train to/from Merced or Reno
Richmond or Emeryville ←→ Merced	Amtrak	2.5	4 times daily
Richmond or Emeryville ←→ Reno	Amtrak (train + bus)	6	3–4 times daily
Merced Amtrak station ←→ Yosemite Valley	YARTS	3	5–6 times daily
Mammoth Lakes ←→ Tuolumne Meadows ←→ Yosemite Valley	YARTS	4	Once daily, in the morning (July, Aug.); Sat.–Sun. only (June, Sept.)
Mammoth Lakes ←→ Tuolumne Meadows	YARTS	2	3 times daily, all in the morning (July, Aug.); Sat.–Sun. only (June, Sept.)
Bishop ←→ Lone Pine	EST	1	2–3 times a day, Mon.–Fri.; no Sat.–Sun. service
Bishop ←→ Mammoth Lakes	EST	1	3 times a day, Mon.–Fri.; no Sat.–Sun. service
Lone Pine ←→ Mammoth Lakes ←→ Reno	EST	5	Once a day, Mon., Tues., Thurs., Fri.
Mammoth Lakes ←→ Lancaster	EST	6	Once a day, Mon., Wed., Fri.
Lancaster ←→ LAX	Antelope Express	2	7 times daily

EST and YARTS Bus Stop Locations

Yosemite Valley   YARTS buses stop at multiple locations, including Curry Village and Yosemite Lodge.

Tuolumne Meadows (Yosemite National Park)   YARTS buses stop at the Tuolumne store.

Lee Vining Southbound EST buses stop at the Chevron station, and northbound EST buses stop at the Caltrans maintenance yard. YARTS buses stop at the Tioga Mobil Mart just south of town.

June Lake EST buses stop at the intersection of US 395 and CA 158. YARTS buses stop at the Rush Creek Trailhead.

Mammoth Lakes EST buses stop at McDonald's (near the east end of Mammoth Lakes), and YARTS buses stop at many locations, including the Mammoth Mountain Inn and Shilo Inn.

Bishop EST buses stop at 1200 North Main Street, the Kmart parking lot.

Big Pine EST buses stop on Main Street, near the center of town.

Independence Southbound EST buses stop at the post office, and northbound EST buses stop at the courthouse.

Lone Pine EST buses stop at the McDonald's at 601 South Main Street.

Charter Services

The businesses and people listed below provide private shuttles between trailheads.

East Side Sierra Shuttle (Paul Fretheim)
760-878-8047 or 760-878-9155
eastsidesierrashuttle.com (based in Independence)

Mt. Whitney Shuttle Service
760-876-1915
mountwhitneyshuttle.com (based in Lone Pine)

Mammoth Taxi
760-937-8294
mammoth-taxi.com

Dave Sheldon
760-876-8232 (based in Lone Pine)

Eastern Sierra Transit Dial-a-Ride
760-873-7173
estransit.com/CMS
Door-to-door van service within the communities of Mammoth Lakes, Bishop, and Lone Pine

Additional information is available at the following websites:
climber.org/data/shuttles.html
groups.yahoo.com/neo/groups/johnmuirtrail/info

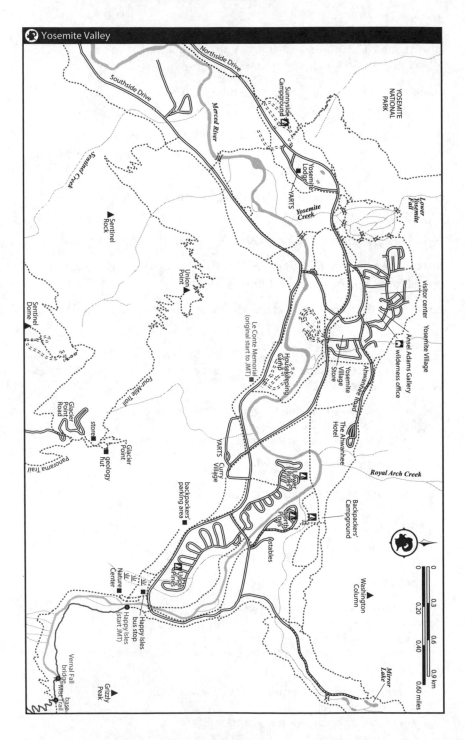

Trailhead Maps

Maps of Yosemite Valley (opposite page), Tuolumne Meadows (page 10), and Lone Pine (page 11) will help orient you at the main trailheads.

Food Resupplies

There are a number of methods to resupply yourself with food along the trail. You can exit the trail to pick up food at a resort, post office, or one of the package-holding services listed below; have someone drive your food to a trailhead (a courier service); or have your food packed into the JMT by stock.

Three Most Commonly Used Resorts

Red's Meadow Resort: Accessed from either the eastern or western Reds Meadow junctions or from Devils Postpile. See the map on page 28 for a detail of trails in the area. **redsmeadow.com**

Vermilion Valley Resort: Accessed from Lake Edison Trail or Lake Edison Ferry, Goodale Pass Trail, Bear Ridge Trail, or Bear Creek Trail. The Lake Edison Ferry costs $12 one-way or $19 round-trip. It usually runs twice daily, leaving the VVR landing at 9 a.m. and 4 p.m., and leaving the ferry wharf on the east side of Lake Edison at 9:45 a.m. and 4:45 p.m. See the table on page 109 for additional information on how best to access VVR, and see pages 34–35 for a map of the area. **edisonlake.com**

Muir Trail Ranch: Accessed from either the northern Muir Trail Ranch cutoff or the southern Muir Trail Ranch cutoff. It is on a spur trail along the trail to Florence Lake. **muirtrailranch.com**

Post Offices

Following is a list of post offices in *some* of the towns along the JMT, in north-to-south order. Unless noted they are open only Monday–Friday. When mailing your package to any of these places, address it to:

[your name]
c/o General Delivery
[name of post office]
[address]
[city], CA [zip code]
HOLD UNTIL [date]

(Continued on page 12)

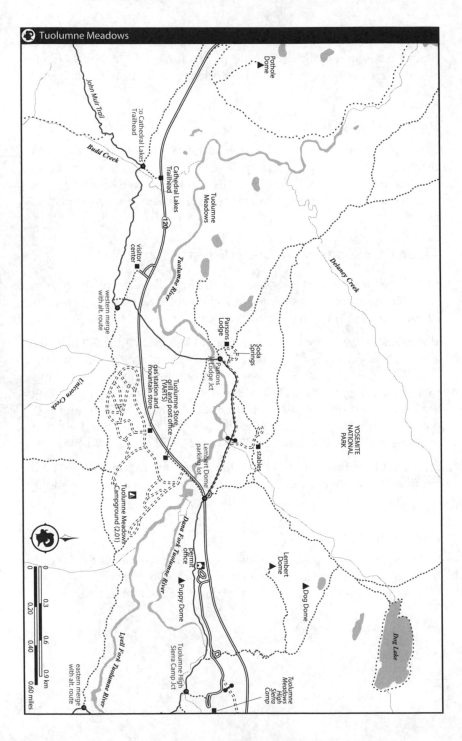

Tuolumne Meadows

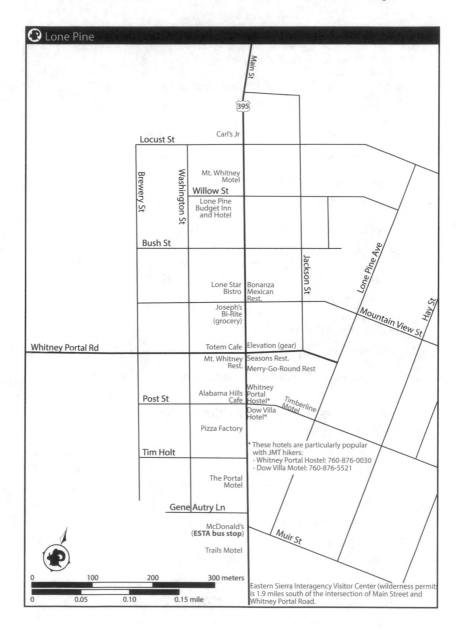

Lone Pine

Main St

395

Locust St   Carl's Jr

Brewery St   Washington St   Mt. Whitney Motel
Willow St
Lone Pine Budget Inn and Hotel

Bush St

Lone Star Bistro   Bonanza Mexican Rest.

Jackson St   Lone Pine Ave

Joseph's Bi-Rite (grocery)

Mountain View St   Hay St

Whitney Portal Rd   Totem Cafe   Elevation (gear)

Mt. Whitney Rest.   Seasons Rest.
Merry-Go-Round Rest

Post St   Alabama Hills Cafe   Whitney Portal Hostel*   Timberline Motel
Dow Villa Hotel*

Pizza Factory

Tim Holt   * These hotels are particularly popular with JMT hikers:
- Whitney Portal Hostel: 760-876-0030
- Dow Villa Motel: 760-876-5521

The Portal Motel

Gene Autry Ln

McDonald's
(ESTA bus stop)

Muir St

Trails Motel

0   100   200   300 meters

0   0.05   0.10   0.15 mile

Eastern Sierra Interagency Visitor Center (wilderness permits) is 1.9 miles south of the intersection of Main Street and Whitney Portal Road.

(Continued from page 9)

Yosemite National Park Post Office
9017 Village Dr.
Yosemite National Park, CA 95389-9998 (open Saturday morning)

Tuolumne Meadows Post Office
14000 CA 120 E
Yosemite National Park, CA 95389-9906 (open Saturday morning)

Mammoth Lakes Post Office
3330 Main St.
Mammoth Lakes, CA 93546-9997

Bishop Post Office
585 W Line St.
Bishop, CA 93514-9998 (open Saturday morning)

Independence Post Office
101 S Edwards St.
Independence, CA 93526-9997

Lone Pine Post Office
121 E Bush St.
Lone Pine, CA 93545-9997

Mono Hot Springs
72000 CA 168
Mono Hot Springs, CA 93642-9800 (open Saturday)

Courier Services, Package-Holding Services, and Pack Resupply

A number of individuals and businesses simplify your food resupplies by allowing you to mail your food to them or by picking up your package from the post office. They will then either drive it to the trailhead for you or hold it for you to pick up outside of post office hours. An alternative option is to have your food carried in by one of the pack stations operating in the region.

East Side Sierra Shuttle (Paul Fretheim)
760-878-8047
eastsidesierrashuttle.com
Paul provides courier and package-holding services.

Mt. Williamson Motel and Base Camp (Cris Chater)
PO Box 128
515 S Edwards St. (US 395)
Independence, CA 93526
760-878-2121
855-787-4333
mtwilliamsonmotel.com
Mt. Williamson Motel provides courier and package-holding services.

Sequoia Kings Pack Trains (Brian and Danica Berner)
PO Box 209
Independence, CA 93526
800-962-0775 or 760-387-2797 (Danica)
bernerspack@yahoo.com
The Berners provide courier, package-holding, and pack resupply services over Kearsarge Pass.

Parchers Resort
5001 S Lake Rd.
Bishop, CA 93514
760-873-4177
parchersresort.net/backpackerservices.htm
Parchers Resort provides package-holding services near the South Lake Trailhead over Bishop Pass.

Rainbow Pack Outfitters (Greg and Ruby Allen)
PO Box 1791
Bishop, CA 93515
760-873-8877
rainbow.zb-net.com
Rainbow Pack Outfitters provides pack resupply services over Bishop Pass.

Cedar Grove Pack Trains (Tim Loverin)
559-565-3464
Cedar Grove Pack Trains provides pack resupply services to Woods Creek or Bubbs Creek.

Waypoints

A GPS-uploadable file with all waypoints given in this book is available on the Wilderness Press website at **bit.ly/JMTgps** and at the John Muir Trail Yahoo Group (**groups.yahoo.com /neo/groups/johnmuirtrail/info**).

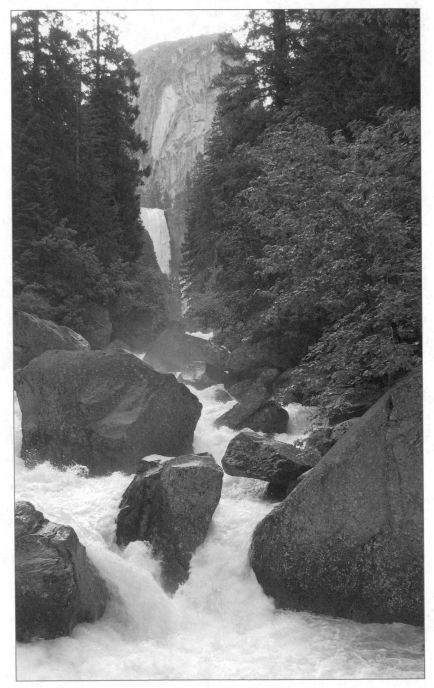

Vernal Fall

TOPOGRAPHIC MAPS

The maps were created from the latest digital elevation models available from the U.S. Geological Survey (USGS) in combination with additional data layers from the USGS, the United States Department of Agriculture, and the National Park Service. The trail data for the JMT and about 75% of the side trails are derived from GPS tracks that I have collected and then edited to more perfectly match the trail as visible on aerial photos available through the USGS (via ExpertGPS) and Google Earth. GPS tracks for a few additional side trails came from other hikers who kindly shared their data with me. The remaining side trails have been traced off USGS topo maps. This section also includes a sketch map of trails in the Devils Postpile and Reds Meadows area.

Map Legend			
●	JMT junction	————	John Muir Trail
▲7.08	JMT campsite	··········	Maintained trail
🏠	Ranger station	········	Unmaintained trail
▲	Summit	═══	Road (paved)
)(	Pass	=======	Road (unpaved)
⬤	Body of water	· — · — ··	National park or forest boundary
❄	Glacier or permanent snowfield	– – – –	Wilderness boundary
⅂⅂	Marsh	⌃2000–	index contours 1000 feet
————	Stream		(contour interval 200 feet)
^^^^^^^^	Ridgeline	⫟	magnetic north 13°05' east of
⊓⊓⊓⊓⊓⊓	Cliffs		geographic north
			1927 North American datum

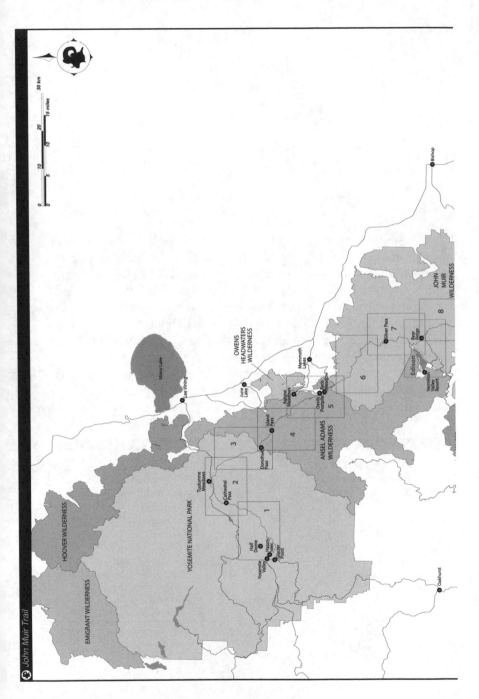

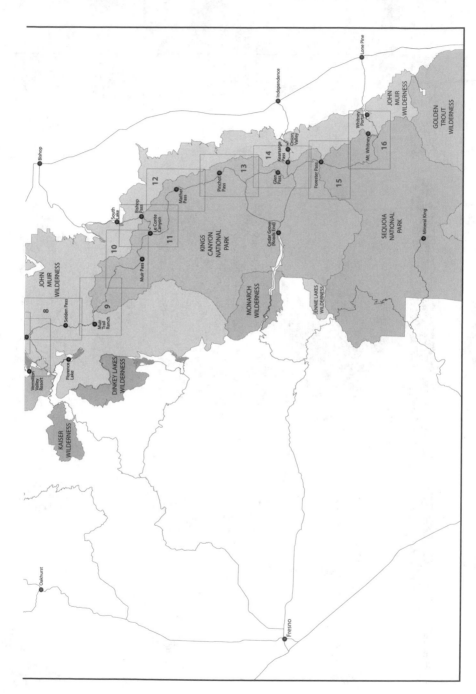

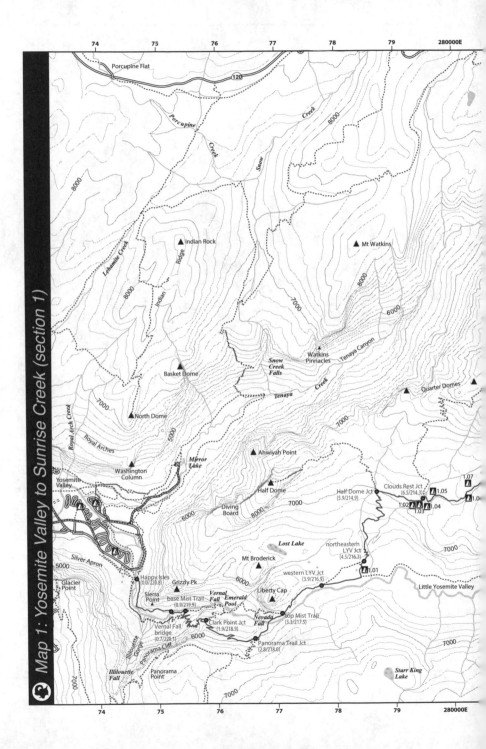

Map 1: Yosemite Valley to Sunrise Creek (section 1)

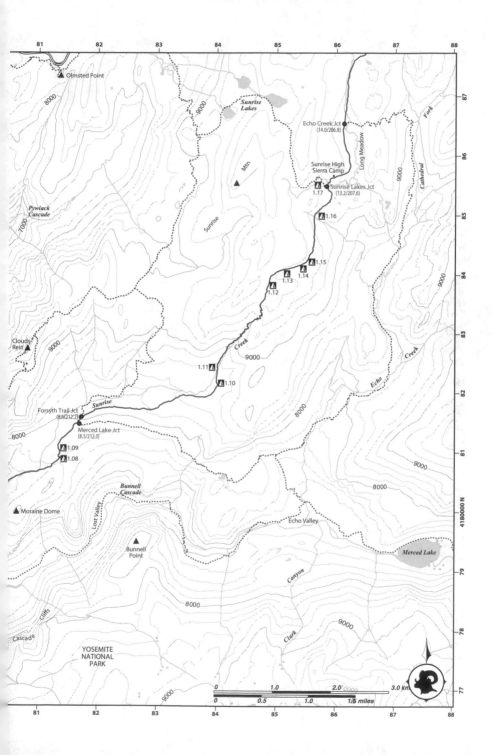

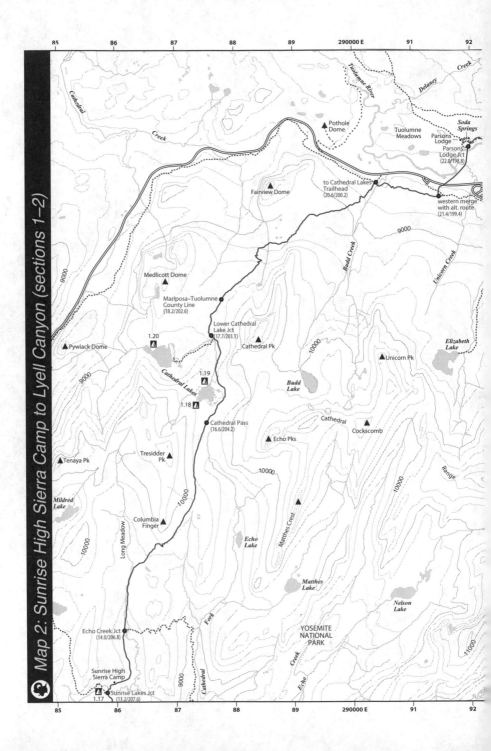

Cathedral Creek

Tuolumne River

Creek

Delaney

Pothole Dome

Tuolumne Meadows

Parsons Lodge

Soda Springs

Parsons Lodge Jct (22.0/198.8)

Fairview Dome

to Cathedral Lakes Trailhead (20.6/200.2)

western merge with alt. route (21.4/199.4)

9000

Budd Creek

Unicorn Creek

Medlicott Dome

Mariposa–Tuolumne County Line (18.2/202.6)

Lower Cathedral Lake Jct (17.7/203.1)

1.20

Cathedral Pk

10000

Elizabeth Lake

Pywiack Dome

Cathedral Lakes

1.19

Unicorn Pk

9000

Budd Lake

1.18

Cathedral

Cockscomb

Cathedral Pass (16.6/204.2)

Echo Pks

Tenaya Pk

Tresidder Pk

10000

Range

10000

Mildred Lake

10000

Columbia Finger

Long Meadow

10000

Echo Lake

Matthes Crest

Matthes Lake

Nelson Lake

11000

Fork

Echo Creek Jct (14.0/206.8)

YOSEMITE NATIONAL PARK

Cathedral

9000

Creek

Echo

Sunrise High Sierra Camp

1.17

Sunrise Lakes Jct (13.2/207.6)

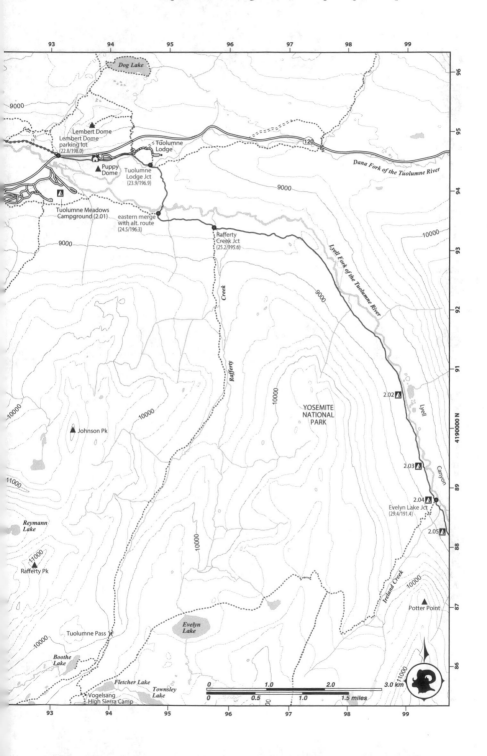

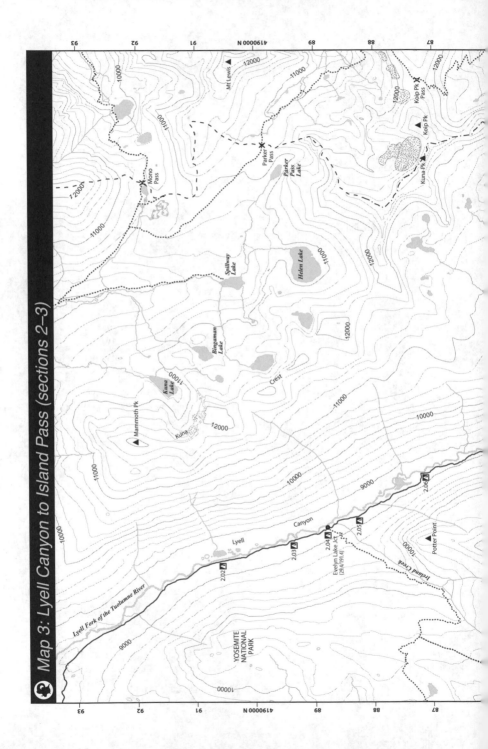

Map 3: Lyell Canyon to Island Pass (sections 2–3)

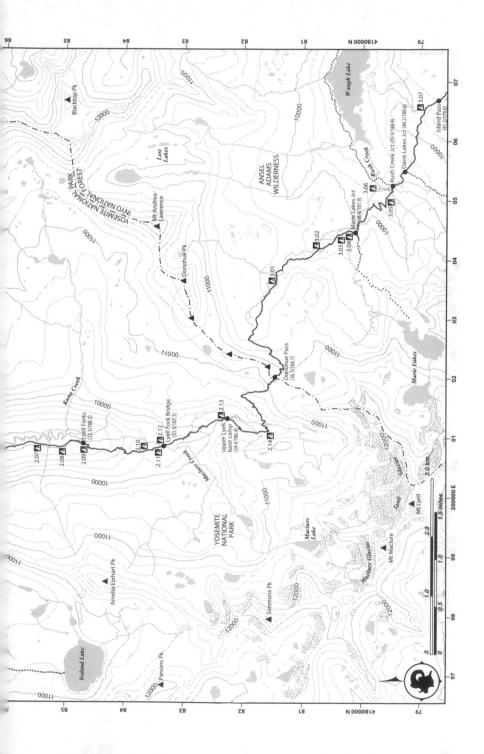

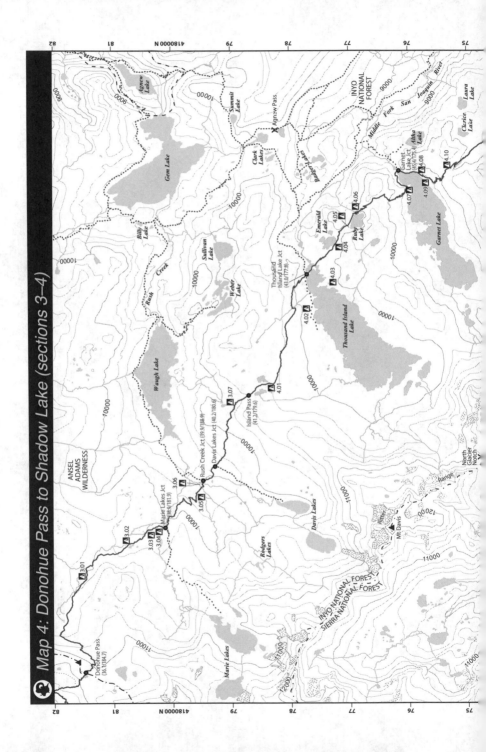

Map 4: Donohue Pass to Shadow Lake (sections 3–4)

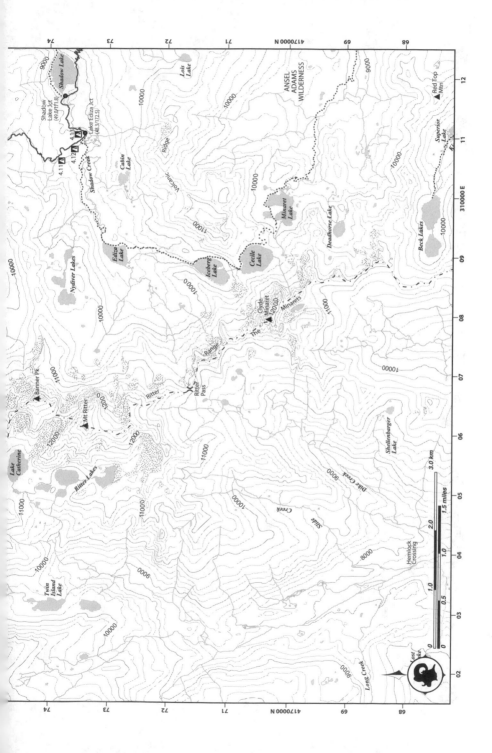

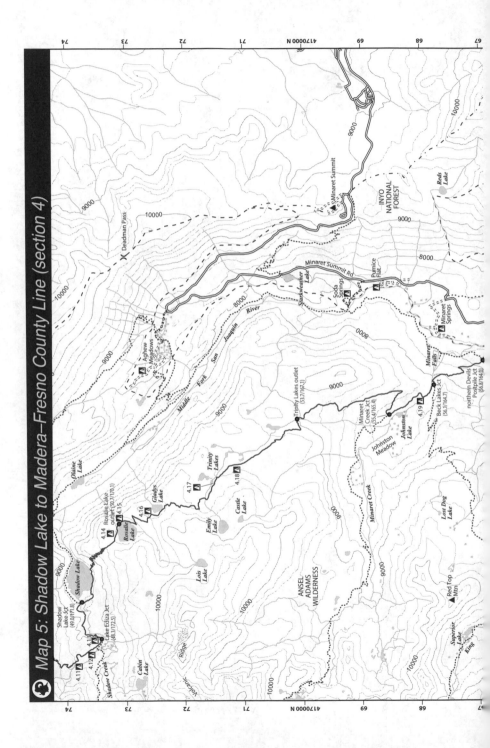

Map 5: Shadow Lake to Madera–Fresno County Line (section 4)

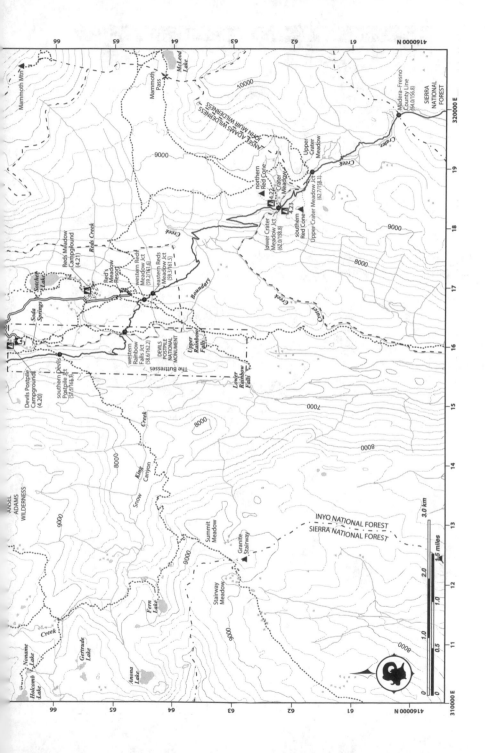

Mammoth Mtn

McLeod Lake

Mammoth Pass

MADERA–FRESNO COUNTY LINE

Madera–Fresno County Line (64.0/156.8)

SIERRA NATIONAL FOREST

10000

9000

ANSEL ADAMS WILDERNESS / JOHN MUIR WILDERNESS

Upper Crater Meadow

northern Red Cone

4.22

Crater Meadow

4.23

Crater Creek

9000

Reds Creek

lower Crater Meadow Jct (62.0/158.8)

southern Red Cone

Upper Crater Meadow Jct (62.7/158.1)

Reds Meadow Campground (4.21)

Red's Meadow Resort

western Reds Meadow Jct (59.2/141.6)

eastern Reds Meadow Jct (59.3/161.5)

9000

8000

Satchet Lake

Boundary

Crater Creek

Soda Springs

western Rainbow Falls Jct (58.6/162.2)

DEVILS POSTPILE NATIONAL MONUMENT

Upper Rainbow Falls

Devils Postpile Campground (4.20)

southern Devils Postpile Jct (57.5/163.1)

The Buttresses

Lower Rainbow Falls

7000

8000

King Creek

8000

8000

ANSEL ADAMS WILDERNESS

Snow Canyon

9000

Summit Meadow

Granite Stairway

INYO NATIONAL FOREST

SIERRA NATIONAL FOREST

3.0 km

1.5 miles

2.0

1.0

Stairway Meadow

9000

Fern Lake

9000

Creek

8000

1.0

0.5

Noname Lake

Gertrude Lake

Anona Lake

Holcomb Lake

0

0

320000 E

N 4160000 N

310000 E

N 4160000 N

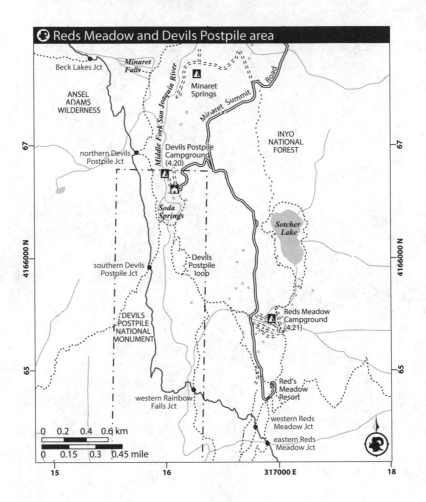

Reds Meadow and Devils Postpile area

Beck Lakes Jct

Minaret Falls

Middle Fork San Joaquin River

Minaret Springs

Minaret Summit

Road

ANSEL ADAMS WILDERNESS

INYO NATIONAL FOREST

northern Devils Postpile Jct

Devils Postpile Campground (4.20)

Soda Springs

Sotcher Lake

southern Devils Postpile Jct

Devils Postpile loop

DEVILS POSTPILE NATIONAL MONUMENT

Reds Meadow Campground (4.21)

Red's Meadow Resort

western Rainbow Falls Jct

western Reds Meadow Jct

eastern Reds Meadow Jct

0   0.2   0.4   0.6 km

0   0.15   0.3   0.45 mile

15   16   317000 E   18

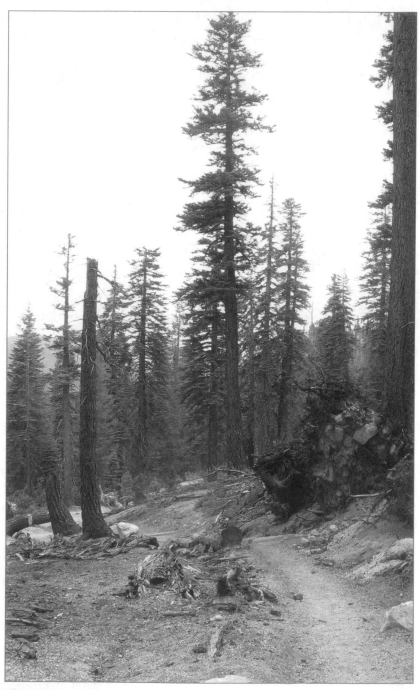

Devils Postpile

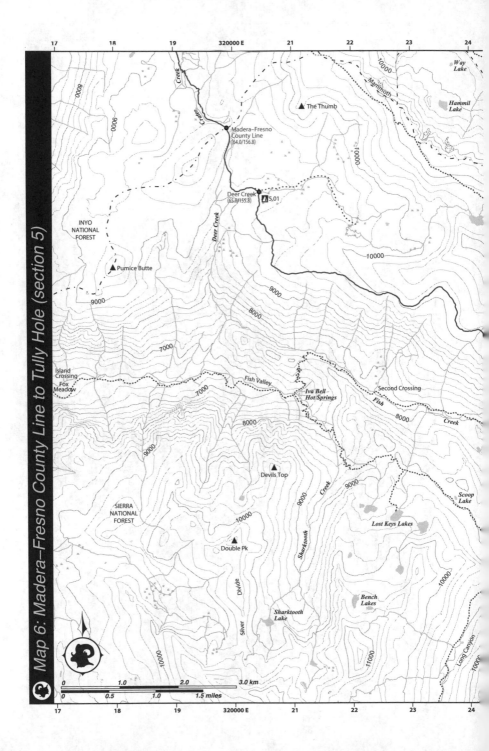

Map 6: Madera–Fresno County Line to Tully Hole (section 5)

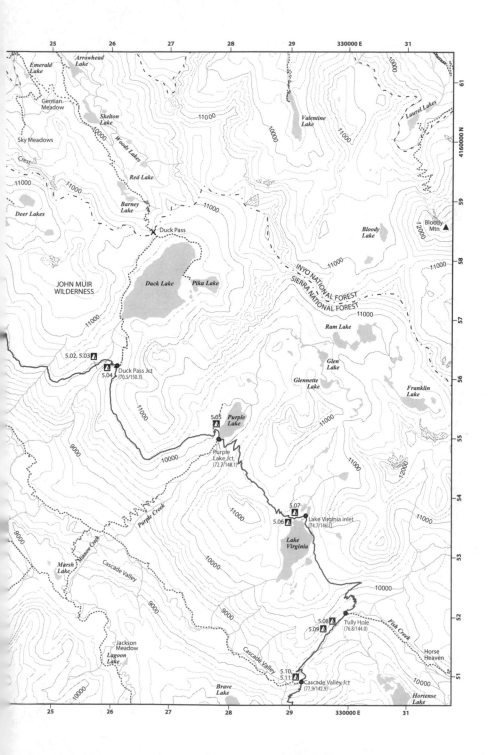

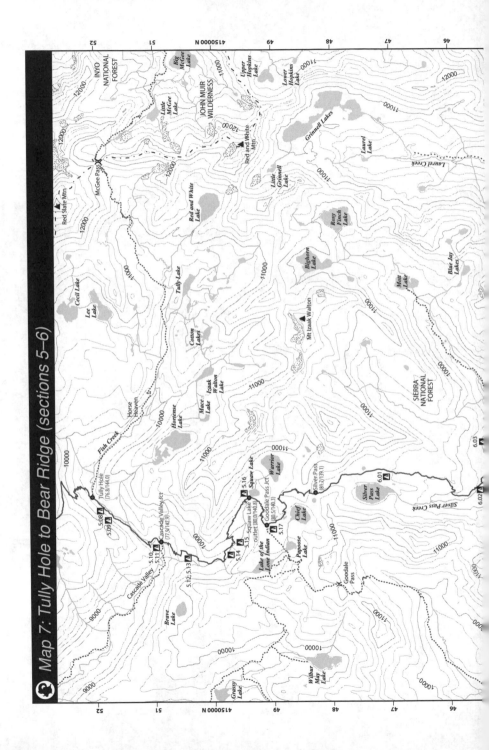

Map 7: Tully Hole to Bear Ridge (sections 5–6)

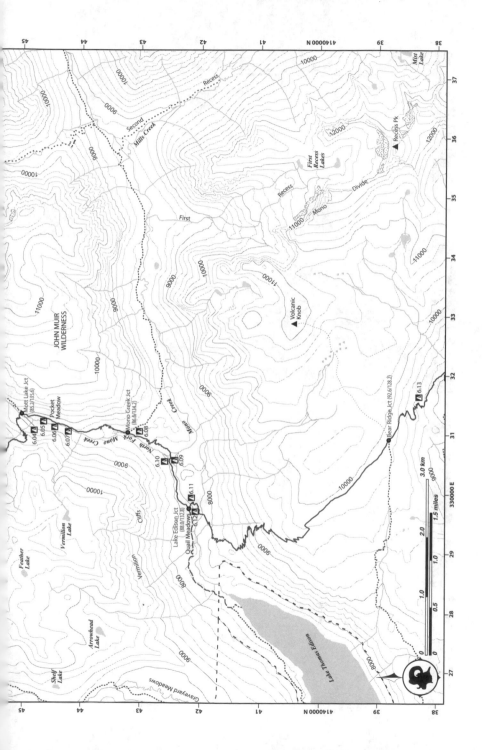

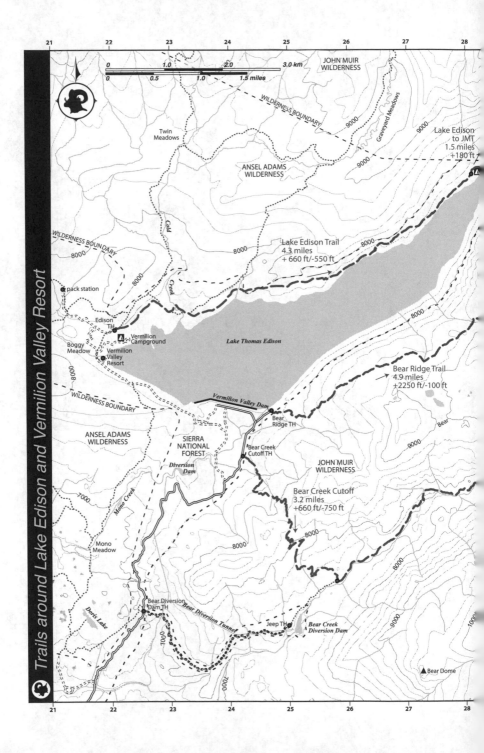

Trails around Lake Edison and Vermilion Valley Resort

JOHN MUIR
WILDERNESS

0   1.0   2.0   3.0 km
0   0.5   1.0   1.5 miles

Twin
Meadows

WILDERNESS BOUNDARY

ANSEL ADAMS
WILDERNESS

Graveyard Meadows

9000

9000

9000

Lake Edison
to JMT
1.5 miles
+180 ft

Cold

Creek

WILDERNESS BOUNDARY

8000

8000

Lake Edison Trail
4.3 miles
+ 660 ft/-550 ft

8000

8000

pack station

Edison
TH

Vermilion
Campground

Boggy
Meadow

Vermilion
Valley
Resort

8000

Lake Thomas Edison

8000

Bear Ridge Trail
4.9 miles
+2250 ft/-100 ft

WILDERNESS BOUNDARY

Vermilion Valley Dam

Bear
Ridge TH

Bear

ANSEL ADAMS
WILDERNESS

SIERRA
NATIONAL
FOREST

Diversion
Dam

Bear Creek
Cutoff TH

9000

JOHN MUIR
WILDERNESS

Mono Creek

7000

Bear Creek Cutoff
3.2 miles
+660 ft/-750 ft

8000

Mono
Meadow

8000

Doris Lake

Bear Diversion
Dam TH

Bear Diversion Tunnel

7000

Jeep TH

Bear Creek
Diversion Dam

9000

1000

7000

Bear Dome

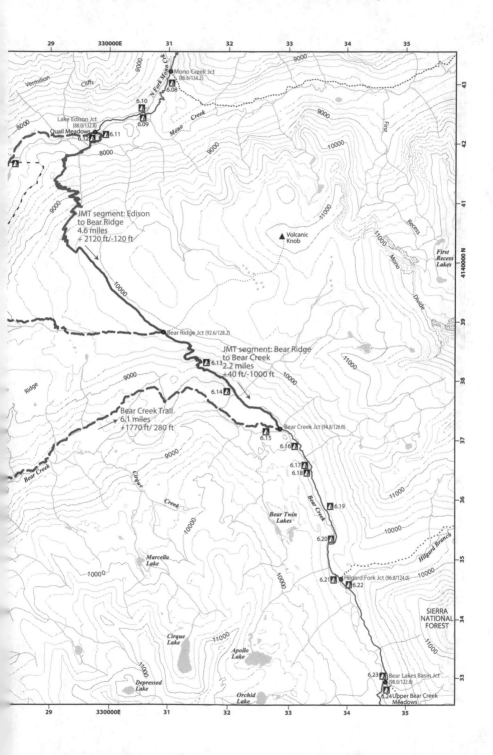

29   330000E   31   32   33   34   35

Vermilion

Cliffs

9000

N Fork Mono Ck

Mono Creek Jct
(86.6/134.2)
6.08

6.10

Lake Edison Jct
(88.0/132.8)
Quail Meadows
6.12 | 6.11

6.09

Mono Creek

8000

8000

9000

9000

9000

10000

First

9000

11000

10000

JMT segment: Edison
to Bear Ridge
4.6 miles
+ 2120 ft/-120 ft

Volcanic
Knob

First
Recess
Lakes

10000

11000

Mono

Recess

414000 N

Divide

Bear Ridge Jct (92.6/128.2)

6.13

JMT segment: Bear Ridge
to Bear Creek
2.2 miles
+40 ft/-1000 ft

Ridge

9000

6.14

10000

11000

Bear Creek Trail
6.1 miles
+1770 ft/ 280 ft

Bear Creek Jct (94.8/126.0)

6.15

6.16

Bear Creek

9000

Cirque

Creek

6.17
6.18

6.19

11000

Bear Twin
Lakes

10000

Marcella
Lake

10000

10000

6.20

Hilgard Branch

10000

6.21 | Hilgard Fork Jct (96.8/124.0)
6.22

Cirque
Lake

11000

SIERRA
NATIONAL
FOREST

Apollo
Lake

10000

11000

11000

Depressed
Lake

Orchid
Lake

6.23 | Bear Lakes Basin Jct
(98.0/122.8)

6.24 Upper Bear Creek
Meadows

Bear Creek

29   330000E   31   32   33   34   35

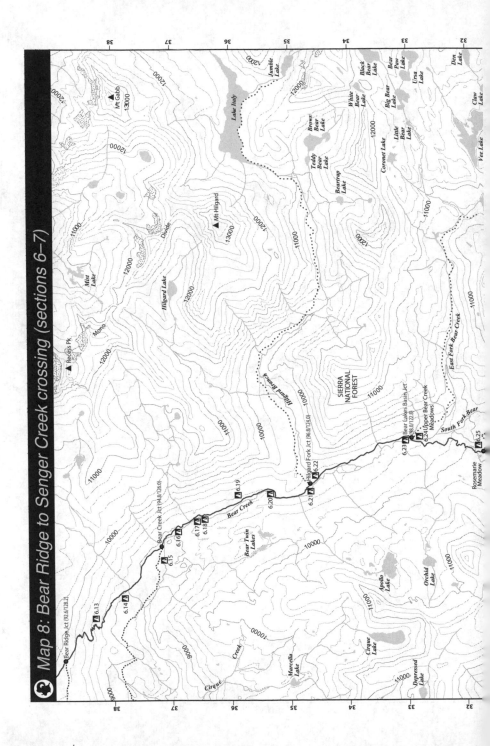

Map 8: Bear Ridge to Senger Creek crossing (sections 6–7)

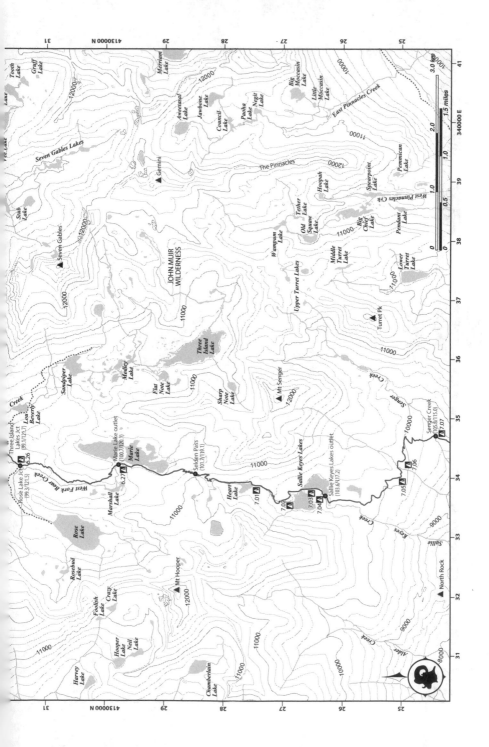

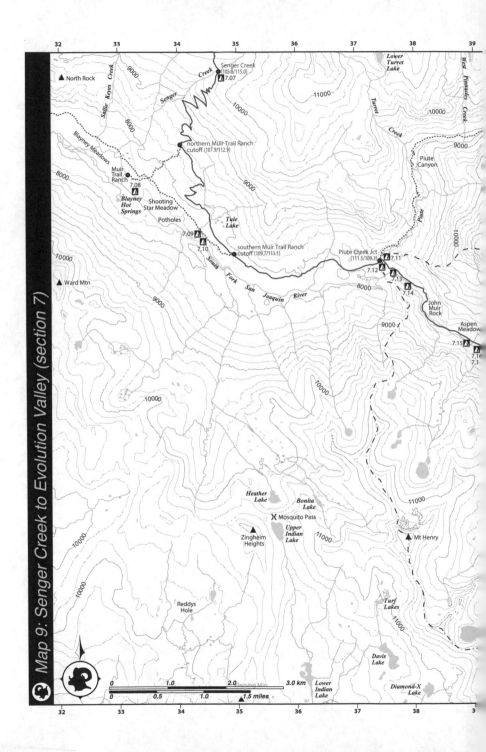

Map 9: Senger Creek to Evolution Valley (section 7)

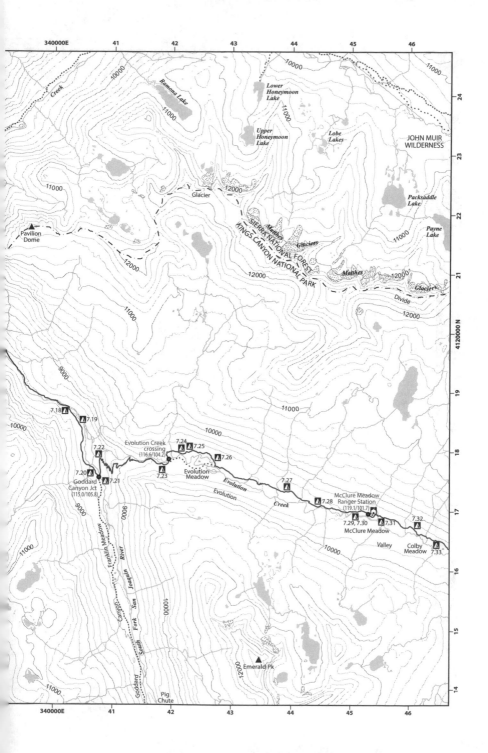

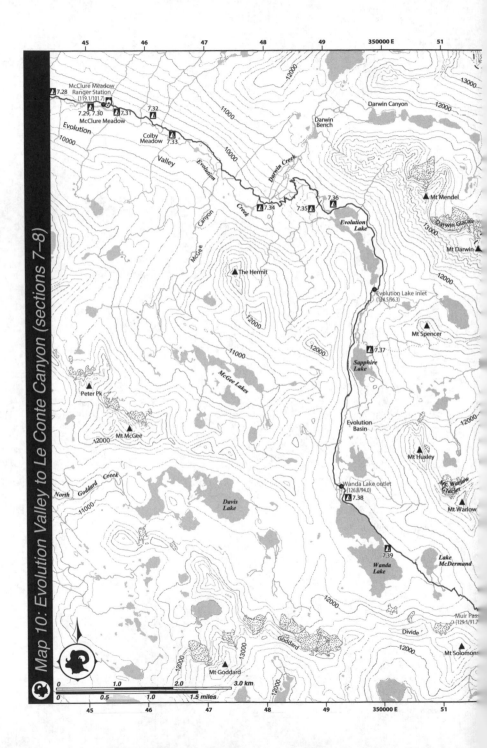

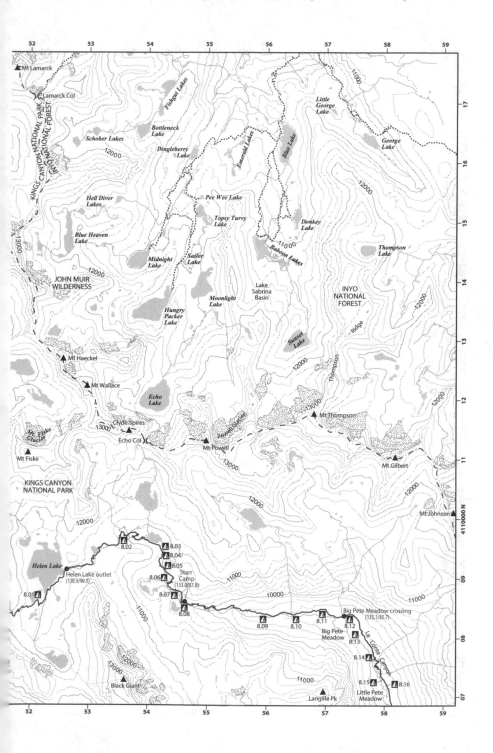

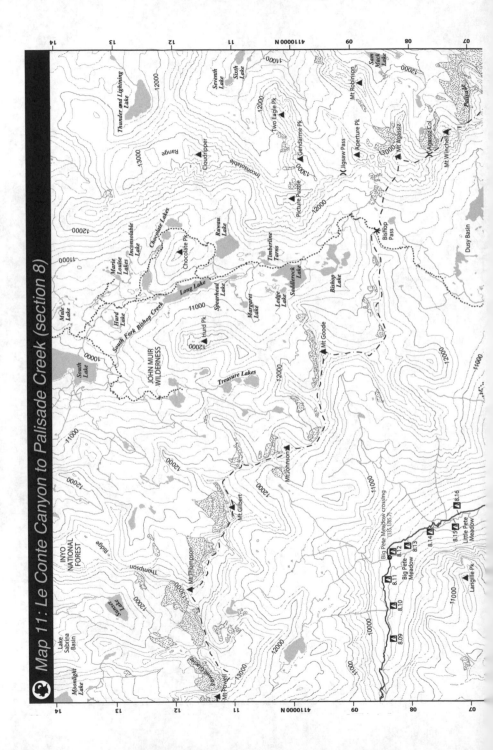

Map 11: Le Conte Canyon to Palisade Creek (section 8)

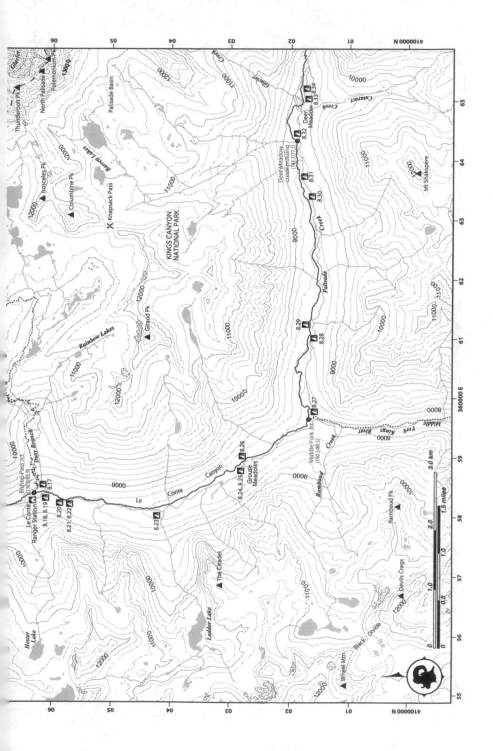

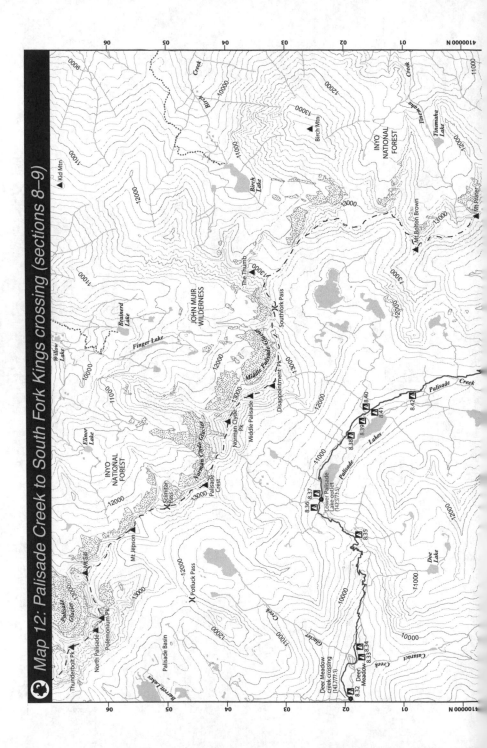

Map 12: Palisade Creek to South Fork Kings crossing (sections 8–9)

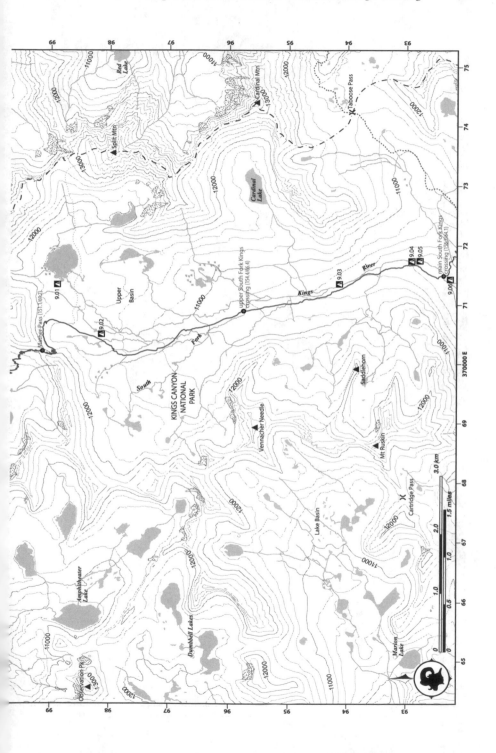

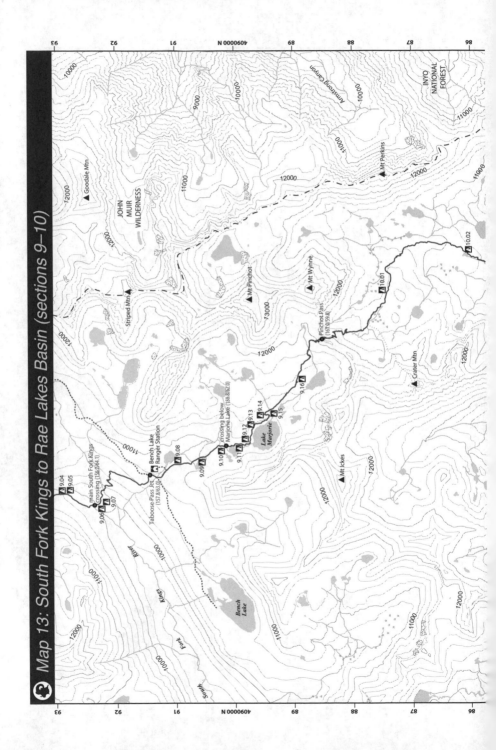

Map 13: South Fork Kings to Rae Lakes Basin (sections 9–10)

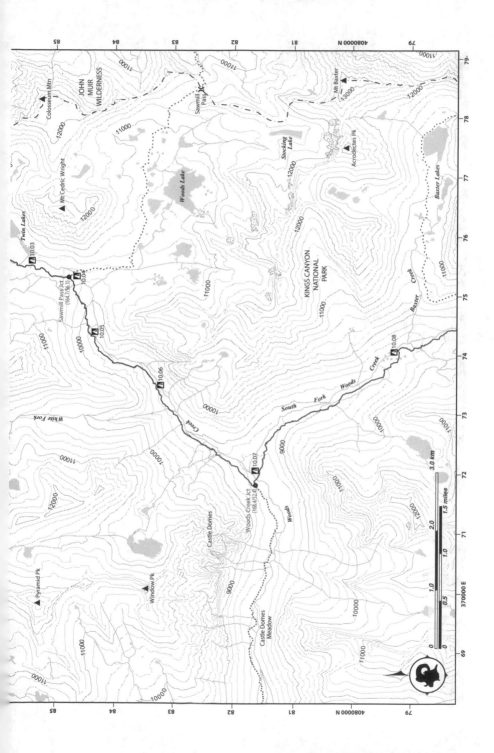

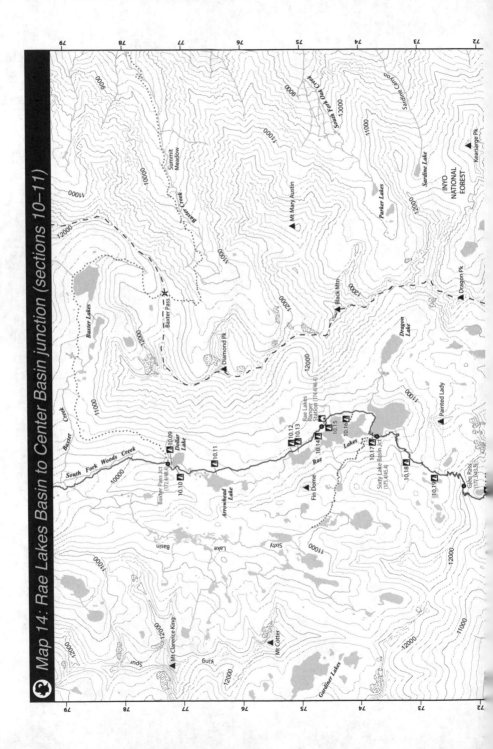

Map 14: Rae Lakes Basin to Center Basin junction (sections 10–11)

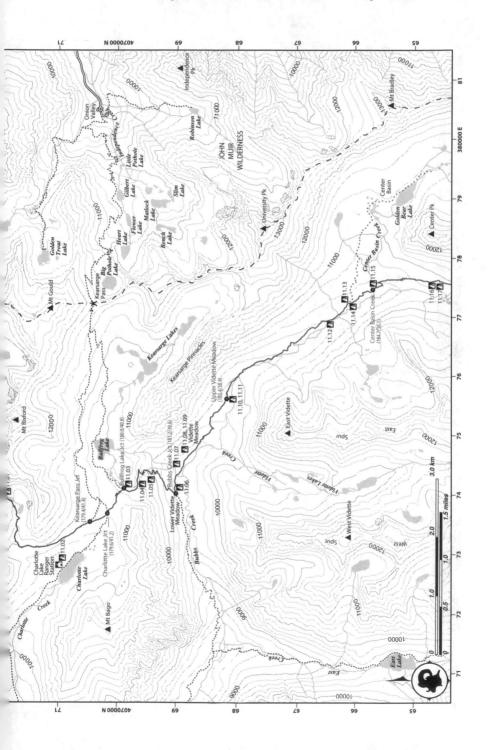

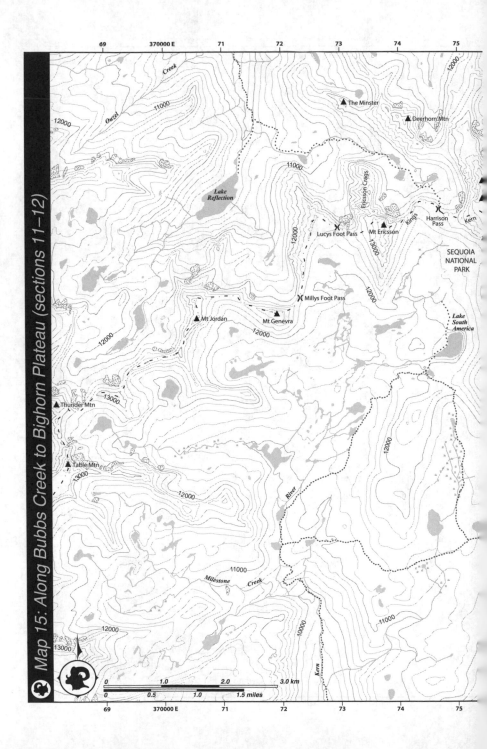

Map 15: Along Bubbs Creek to Bighorn Plateau (sections 11–12)

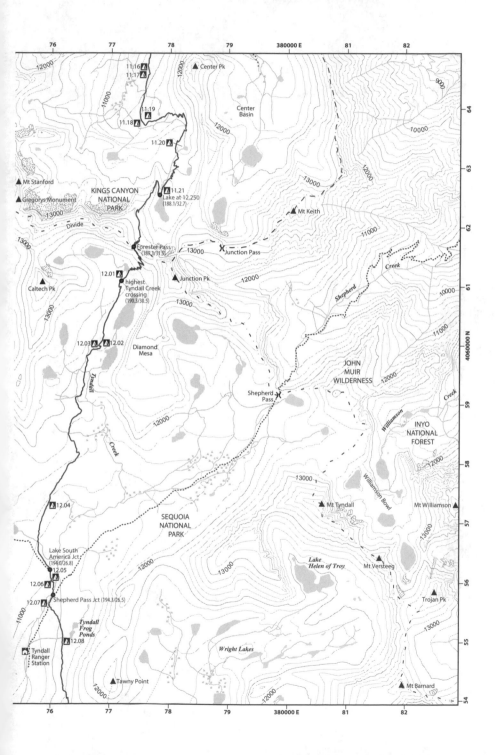

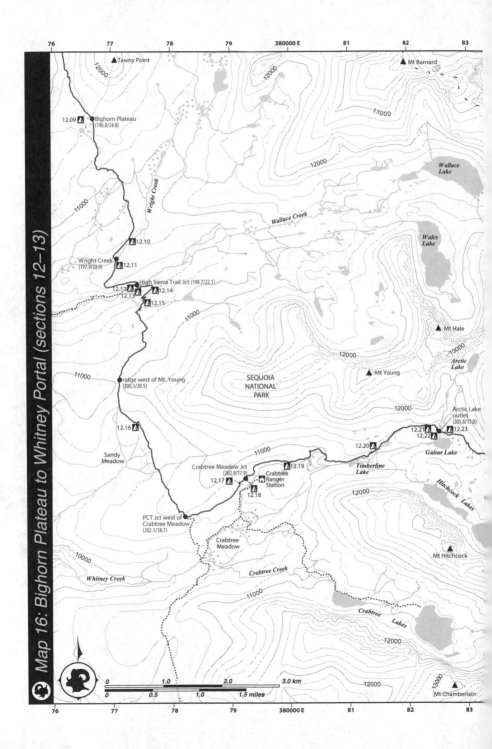

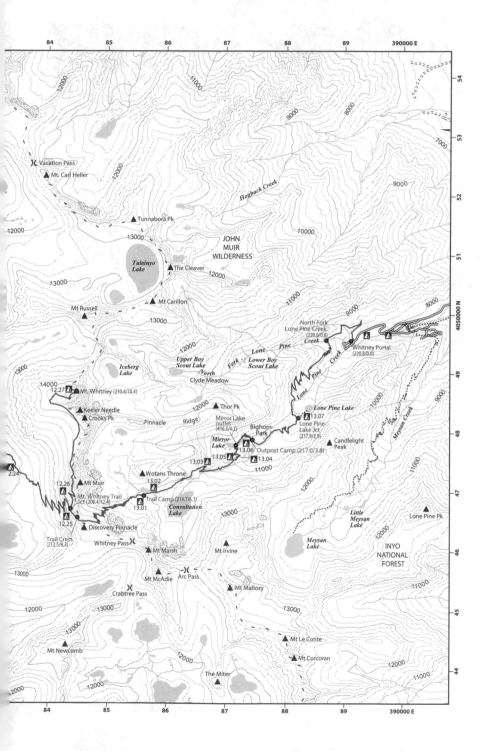

84   85   86   87   88   89   390000 E

12000

11000

9000

8000

7000

)(Vacation Pass
▲ Mt. Carl Heller

Hogback Creek

9000

12000

12000

▲ Tunnabora Pk

13000

JOHN
MUIR
WILDERNESS

10000

12000

Tulainyo
Lake

▲ The Cleaver

12000

13000

11000

13000

▲ Mt Carillon

North Fork
Lone Pine Creek
(220.0/0.8)
Creek

9000

8000

Mt Russell
▲

13000

Whitney Portal
(220.8/0.0)

14000

Iceberg
Lake

Upper Boy
Scout Lake

Lone   Pine   Creek

Fork

Lower Boy
Scout Lake

North
Clyde Meadow

Lone Pine Creek

Meysan Creek

12.27 ▲ Mt. Whitney (210.4/10.4)

▲ Thor Pk

Lone Pine Lake

10000

9000

▲ Keeler Needle
▲ Crooks Pk

Pinnacle   Ridge

Mirror Lake
outlet
(416.6/4.2)

13.07
Lone Pine
Lake Jct
(217.9/2.9)

Candlelight
Peak

12000

Bighorn
Park

Mirror
Lake

2.24

12.26 ▲ Mt Muir

Wotans Throne
13.02

13.06

13.05

13.03

Outpost Camp (217.0/3.8)

13.04

11000

Little
Meysan
Lake

Lone Pine Pk
▲

11000

Mt. Whitney Trail
Jct (208.4/12.4)

Trail Camp (214.7/6.1)

13.01

Consultation
Lake

13000

12.25 ▲ Discovery Pinnacle

Meysan
Lake

INYO
NATIONAL
FOREST

Trail Crest
(212.5/8.3)

Whitney Pass)(

▲ Mt Marsh

▲ Mt Irvine

13000

12000

)(Arc Pass

13000

11000

▲ Mt McAdie

)(Crabtree Pass

▲ Mt Mallory

12000

13000

13000

▲ Mt Le Conte

▲ Mt Corcoran

12000

11000

▲ Mt Newcomb

12000

The Miter

12000

12000

84   85   86   87   88   89   390000 E

54

53

52

51

4050000 N

49

48

47

46

45

44

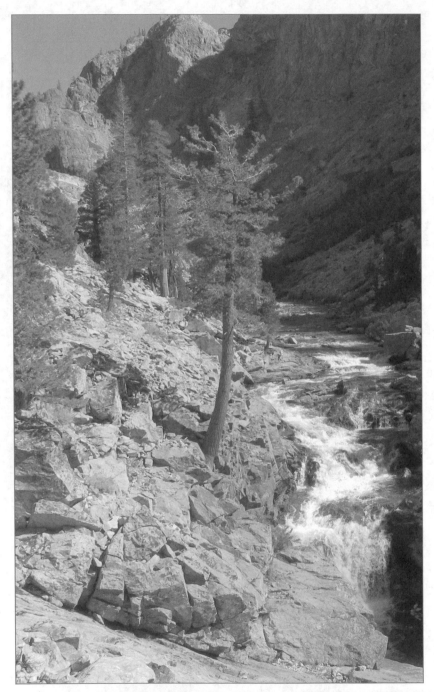

The South Fork of the San Joaquin River tumbling through Goddard Canyon

YOSEMITE VALLEY TO WHITNEY PORTAL

Section 1.

Happy Isles to Tuolumne–Mariposa County Line: Merced River (16.6 miles)

LOCATION	ELEVATION	DISTANCE FROM PREVIOUS POINT	N-S	S-N	UTM COORDINATES
Happy Isles mileage sign	4,040'	—	0.0	220.8	11S 274619E 4178853N
Vernal Fall bridge	4,400'	0.7	0.7	220.1	11S 275203E 4178293N
Mist Trail junction	4,530'	0.2	0.9	219.9	11S 275439E 4178311N
Clark Point junction	5,490'	1.0	1.9	218.9	11S 275776E 4178159N
Panorama Trail junction	6,020'	0.9	2.8	218.0	11S 276619E 4177842N
Nevada Fall junction	6,000'	0.5	3.3	217.5	11S 277075E 4178261N
western Little Yosemite Valley junction	6,110'	0.6	3.9	216.9	11S 277750E 4178733N
northeastern Little Yosemite Valley junction	6,130'	0.6	4.5	216.3	11S 278460E 4179141N
Half Dome junction	6,980'	1.4	5.9	214.9	11S 278685E 4180304N
Clouds Rest junction	7,160'	0.6	6.5	214.3	11S 279499E 4180189N
Merced Lake junction	7,950'	2.0	8.5	212.3	11S 281696E 4181478N
Forsyth Trail junction	8,010'	0.1	8.6	212.2	11S 281730E 4181595N
Sunrise Lakes junction	9,310'	4.6	13.2	207.6	11S 285842E 4185489N
Echo Creek junction	9,310'	0.8	14.0	206.8	11S 286129E 4186546N
Cathedral Pass	9,700'	2.6	16.6	204.2	11S 287532E 4190048N
Lower Cathedral Lake junction	9,430'	1.1	17.7	203.1	11S 287620E 4191522N
Mariposa–Tuolumne County Line	9,570'	0.5	18.2	202.6	11S 287789E 4192140N

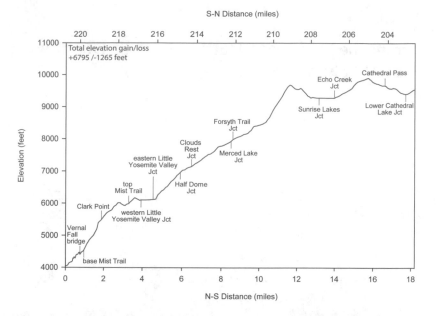

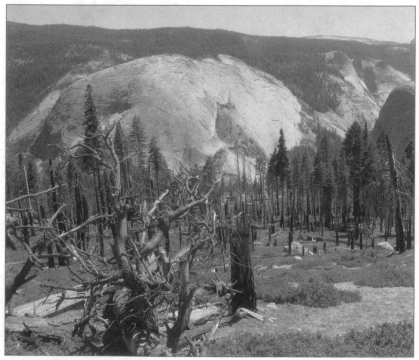

View south to the Merced River Canyon from Sunrise Creek

Section 2.

Tuolumne–Mariposa County Line to Donohue Pass: Tuolumne River (17.9 miles)

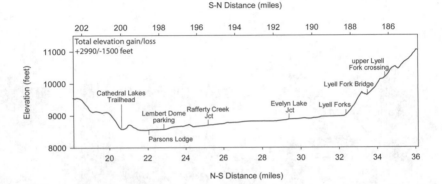

S-N Distance (miles)

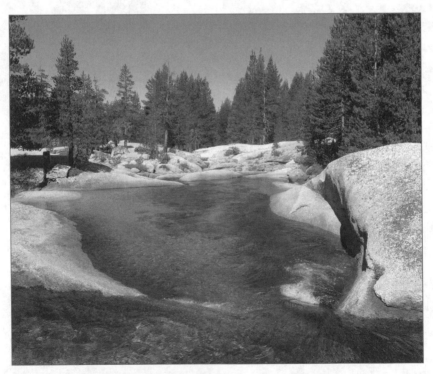

Lyell Fork of the Tuolumne River

LOCATION	ELEVATION	DISTANCE FROM PREVIOUS POINT	N-S	S-N	UTM COORDINATES
Mariposa–Tuolumne County Line	9,570'	—	18.2	202.6	11S 287789E 4192140N
trail to Cathedral Lakes Trailhead	8,600'	2.4	20.6	200.2	11S 290409E 4194106N
western merge with Tuolumne perimeter trail	8,630'	0.8	21.4	199.4	11S 291480E 4193871N
Parsons Lodge junction	8,560'	0.6	22.0	198.8	11S 291982E 4194705N
Lembert Dome parking lot	8,590'	0.8	22.8	198.0	11S 293123E 4194590N
Tuolumne Meadows Lodge junction	8,680'	1.1	23.9	196.9	11S 294682E 4194429N
eastern merge with Tuolumne perimeter trail	8,670'	0.6	24.5	196.3	11S 294819E 4193619N
Rafferty Creek junction	8,720'	0.7	25.2	195.6	11S 295742E 4193386N
Evelyn Lake junction	8,900'	4.2	29.4	191.4	11S 299493E 4188811N
start of climb from Lyell Canyon (Lyell Forks)	9,020'	2.9	32.3	188.5	11S 300899E 4184697N
Lyell Fork Bridge	9,650'	1.2	33.5	187.3	11S 300863E 4183358N
second Lyell Fork crossing	10,190'	0.9	34.4	186.4	11S 301325E 4182269N
Donohue Pass	11,060'	1.7	36.1	184.7	11S 302025E 4181480N

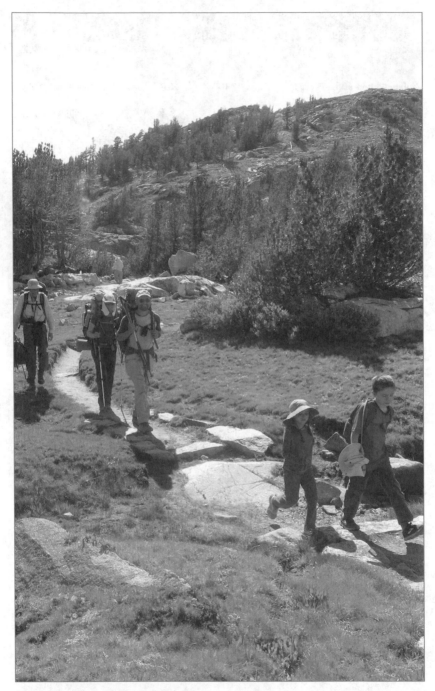

Cresting the top of Island Pass

Section 3.

Donohue Pass to Island Pass: Rush Creek (5.1 miles)

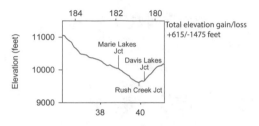

S-N Distance (miles)

LOCATION	ELEVATION	DISTANCE FROM PREVIOUS POINT	N-S	S-N	UTM COORDINATES
Donohue Pass	11,060'	—	36.1	184.7	11S 302025E 4181480N
Marie Lakes junction	10,050'	2.8	38.9	181.9	11S 304468E 4180130N
Rush Creek junction	9,640'	1.0	39.9	180.9	11S 305247E 4179506N
Davis Lakes junction	9,690'	0.3	40.2	180.6	11S 305493E 4179290N
Island Pass	10,200'	1.0	41.2	179.6	11S 306696E 4178711N

Section 4.

Island Pass to Madera–Fresno County Line: Middle Fork of the San Joaquin River (22.8 miles)

LOCATION	ELEVATION	DISTANCE FROM PREVIOUS POINT	N–S	S–N	UTM COORDINATES
Island Pass	10,200'	—	41.2	179.6	11S 306696E 4178711N
Thousand Island Lake junction	9,830'	1.8	43.0	177.8	11S 308733E 4177711N
Garnet Lake junction	9,690'	2.4	45.4	175.4	11S 310473E 4176161N
Lake Ediza junction	9,000'	2.9	48.3	172.5	11S 311074E 4173429N
Shadow Lake junction	8,780'	0.7	49.0	171.8	11S 311695E 4173755N
Rosalie Lake outlet	9,350'	1.7	50.7	170.1	11S 313013E 4173125N
Trinity Lakes outlet crossing	8,990'	3.0	53.7	167.1	11S 314766E 4170105N
Minaret Creek junction (Johnston Meadow)	8,120'	1.7	55.4	165.4	11S 314836E 4168536N
Beck Lakes junction	8,080'	0.7	56.1	164.7	11S 315344E 4167773N
northern Devils Postpile junction	7,680'	0.7	56.8	164.0	11S 315738E 4166946N
southern Devils Postpile junction	7,710'	0.7	57.5	163.3	11S 315861E 4165921N
western Rainbow Falls junction	7,460'	1.1	58.6	162.2	11S 316246E 4164827N
western Reds Meadow junction	7,640'	0.6	59.2	161.6	11S 316792E 4164496N
eastern Reds Meadow junction	7,710'	0.1	59.3	161.5	11S 316898E 4164358N
lower Crater Meadow junction (Mammoth Pass)	8,650'	2.7	62.0	158.8	11S 318340E 4162258N
upper Crater Meadow junction	8,910'	0.7	62.7	158.1	11S 318941E 4161689N
Madera–Fresno County Line	9,210'	1.3	64.0	156.8	11S 319942E 4160144N

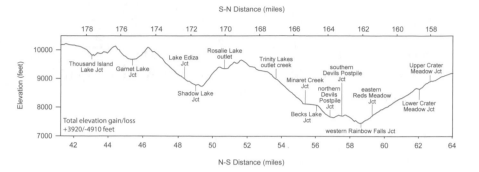

S-N Distance (miles)

Thousand Island Lake Jct
Garnet Lake Jct
Lake Ediza Jct
Rosalie Lake outlet
Trinity Lakes outlet creek
Shadow Lake Jct
Minaret Creek Jct
northern Devils Postpile Jct
southern Devils Postpile Jct
eastern Reds Meadow Jct
Upper Crater Meadow Jct
Becks Lake Jct
Lower Crater Meadow Jct
western Rainbow Falls Jct

Total elevation gain/loss
+3920/-4910 feet

N-S Distance (miles)

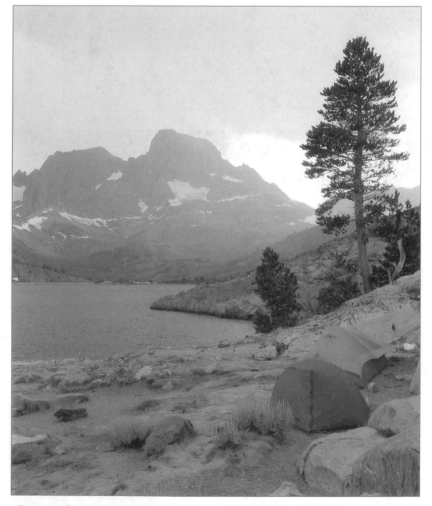

Camp at Garnet Lake with Mt. Ritter and Banner Peak behind

Section 5.

Madera–Fresno County Line to Silver Pass: Fish Creek Fork of the Middle Fork of the San Joaquin River (17.7 miles)

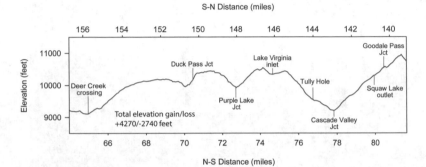

LOCATION	ELEVATION	DISTANCE FROM PREVIOUS POINT	N-S	S-N	UTM COORDINATES
Madera–Fresno County Line	9,210'	—	64.0	156.8	11S 319942E 4160144N
Deer Creek	9,100'	1.0	65.0	155.8	11S 320460E 4159139N
Duck Pass junction	10,160'	5.5	70.5	150.3	11S 326107E 4156217N
Purple Lake trail junction	9,940'	2.2	72.7	148.1	11S 327817E 4154979N
Lake Virginia inlet crossing	10,330'	2.0	74.7	146.1	11S 329263E 4153696N
Tully Hole (McGee Pass junction)	9,540'	2.1	76.8	144.0	11S 329961E 4152066N
Cascade Valley (Fish Creek) junction	9,190'	1.1	77.9	142.9	11S 329202E 4150912N
Squaw Lake outlet	10,290'	2.1	80.0	140.8	11S 329933E 4149416N
Goodale Pass junction	10,540'	0.5	80.5	140.3	11S 329463E 4149123N
Silver Pass	10,740'	1.2	81.7	139.1	11S 330013E 4148295N

Section 6.

Silver Pass to Selden Pass: Mono and Bear Creeks (20.0 miles)

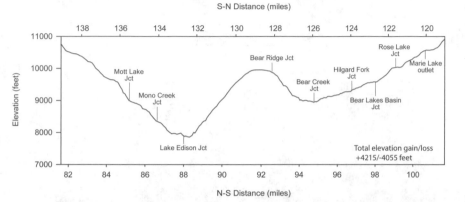

LOCATION	ELEVATION	DISTANCE FROM PREVIOUS POINT	N-S	S-N	UTM COORDINATES
Silver Pass	10,740'	—	81.7	139.1	11S 330013E 4148295N
Mott Lake junction	8,990'	3.5	85.2	135.6	11S 331344E 4145016N
Mono Creek junction	8,350'	1.4	86.6	134.2	11S 331025E 4143220N
Lake Edison (Quail Meadows) junction	7,900'	1.4	88.0	132.8	11S 329749E 4142183N
Bear Ridge junction	9,870'	4.6	92.6	128.2	11S 330920E 4138825N
Bear Creek junction	8,940'	2.2	94.8	126.0	11S 332846E 4137180N
Hilgard Fork junction	9,320'	2.0	96.8	124.0	11S 333894E 4134670N
Bear Lakes Basin junction	9,580'	1.2	98.0	122.8	11S 334658E 4132945N
Three Island Lake junction	10,020'	1.1	99.1	121.7	11S 334430E 4131717N
Rose Lake junction	10,030'	0.2	99.3	121.5	11S 334188E 4131442N
Marie Lake outlet	10,550'	1.4	100.7	120.1	11S 334212E 4129777N
Selden Pass	10,900'	1.0	101.7	119.1	11S 334059E 4128480N

Section 7.

Selden Pass to Muir Pass: South Fork of the San Joaquin River (27.4 miles)

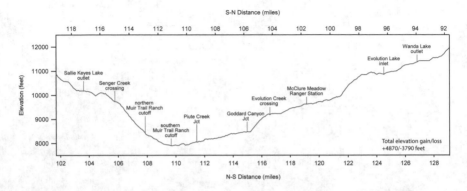

LOCATION	ELEVATION	DISTANCE FROM PREVIOUS POINT	N-S	S-N	UTM COORDINATES
Selden Pass	10,900'	—	101.7	119.1	11S 334059E 4128480N
Sallie Keyes outlet crossing	10,180'	1.9	103.6	117.2	11S 333700E 4126292N
Senger Creek	9,740'	2.2	105.8	115.0	11S 334732E 4124433N
northern Muir Trail Ranch cutoff	8,410'	2.1	107.9	112.9	11S 334050E 4123185N
southern Muir Trail Ranch cutoff	7,900'	1.8	109.7	111.1	11S 334958E 4121342N
Piute Creek junction	8,050'	1.8	111.5	109.3	11S 337416E 4121220N
Goddard Canyon junction	8,480'	3.5	115.0	105.8	11S 340763E 4117572N
Evolution Creek wade	9,190'	1.6	116.6	104.2	11S 341942E 4117874N
McClure Meadow Ranger Station	9,630'	2.5	119.1	101.7	11S 345302E 4116963N
Evolution Lake inlet	10,860'	5.4	124.5	96.3	11S 349857E 4113827N
Wanda Lake outlet	11,380'	2.3	126.8	94.0	11S 349280E 4110505N
Muir Pass	11,980'	2.3	129.1	91.7	11S 351621E 4108409N

Section 8.

Muir Pass to Mather Pass: Middle Fork of the Kings River (22.0 miles)

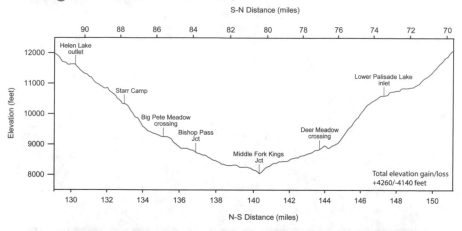

LOCATION	ELEVATION	DISTANCE FROM PREVIOUS POINT	N-S	S-N	UTM COORDINATES
Muir Pass	11,980'	—	129.1	91.7	11S 351621E 4108409N
Helen Lake outlet	11,630'	1.2	130.3	90.5	11S 352635E 4109144N
Starr Camp	10,320	2.7	133.0	87.8	11S 354628E 4108611N
Big Pete Meadow creek crossing	9,240'	2.1	135.1	85.7	11S 357317E 4108373N
Bishop Pass junction	8,740'	1.8	136.9	83.9	11S 358394E 4106307N
Middle Fork junction	8,030'	3.4	140.3	80.5	11S 359641E 4101704N
Deer Meadow creek crossing	8,830'	3.4	143.7	77.1	11S 364332E 4101910N
Lower Palisade Lake outlet	10,600'	3.6	147.3	73.5	11S 367700E 4102388N
Mather Pass	12,100'	3.8	151.1	69.7	11S 370213E 4099138N

Section 9.

Mather Pass to Pinchot Pass: South Fork of the Kings River (9.9 miles)

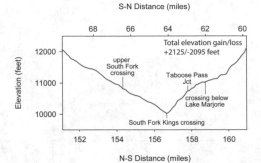

LOCATION	ELEVATION	DISTANCE FROM PREVIOUS POINT	N-S	S-N	UTM COORDINATES
Mather Pass	12,100'	—	151.1	69.7	11S 370213E 4099138N
South Fork Kings crossing at the base of Upper Basin	10,830'	3.3	154.4	66.4	11S 370891E 4095758N
main South Fork Kings crossing	10,040'	2.3	156.7	64.1	11S 371500E 4092362N
Taboose Pass junction	10,760'	1.1	157.8	63.0	11S 371999E 4091444N
crossing below Marjorie Lake	11,050'	1.0	158.8	62.0	11S 372485E 4090166N
Pinchot Pass	12,130'	2.2	161.0	59.8	11S 374287E 4088510N

Section 10.

Pinchot Pass to Glen Pass: Woods Creek Fork of the Kings River (16.3 miles)

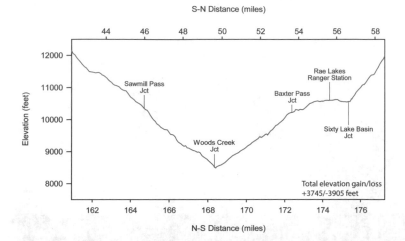

LOCATION	ELEVATION	DISTANCE FROM PREVIOUS POINT	N-S	S-N	UTM COORDINATES
Pinchot Pass	12,130'	—	161.0	59.8	11S 374287E 4088510N
Sawmill Pass junction	10,350'	3.7	164.7	56.1	11S 375315E 4084786N
Woods Creek junction	8,510'	3.7	168.4	52.4	11S 371808E 4081636N
Baxter Pass junction	10,220'	4.0	172.4	48.4	11S 374516E 4077254N
Rae Lakes Ranger Station junction	10,590'	2.0	174.4	46.4	11S 375128E 4074656N
Sixty Lake Basin junction	10,560'	1.0	175.4	45.4	11S 374963E 4073712N
Glen Pass	11,970'	1.9	177.3	43.5	11S 374120E 4072254N

Section 11.

Glen Pass to Forester Pass: Bubbs Creek Fork of the Kings River (12.0 miles)

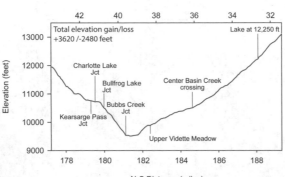

LOCATION	ELEVATION	DISTANCE FROM PREVIOUS POINT	N-S	S-N	UTM COORDINATES
Glen Pass	11,970'	—	177.3	43.5	11S 374120E 4072254N
Kearsarge Pass junction	10,770'	2.1	179.4	41.4	11S 373545E 4070469N
Charlotte Lake junction	10,740'	0.2	179.6	41.2	11S 373685E 4070166N
Bullfrog Lake junction	10,520'	0.4	180.0	40.8	11S 374109E 4069887N
Bubbs Creek junction (Lower Vidette Meadow)	9,550'	1.2	181.2	39.6	11S 374026E 4069006N
Upper Vidette Meadow food box	9,910'	1.2	182.4	38.4	11S 375616E 4068174N
Center Basin Creek	10,530'	2.3	184.7	36.1	11S 377469E 4065704N
Lake at 12,250 feet	12,240'	3.4	188.1	32.7	11S 377813E 4062539N
Forester Pass	13,110'	1.2	189.3	31.5	11S 377379E 4061665N

Section 12.

Forester Pass to Trail Crest:
Kern River (23.2 miles)

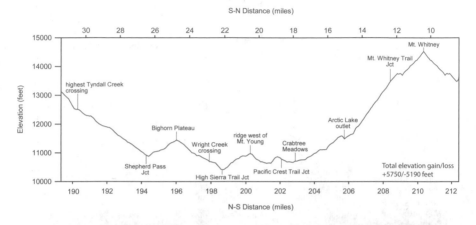

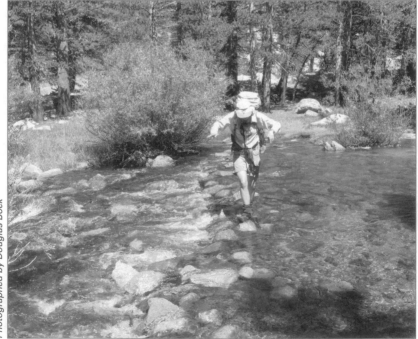

Photographed by Douglas Bock

Wallace Creek crossing

LOCATION	ELEVATION	DISTANCE FROM PREVIOUS POINT	N-S	S-N	UTM COORDINATES
Forester Pass	13,110'	—	189.3	31.5	11S 377379E 4061665N
highest Tyndall Creek crossing	12,500'	1.0	190.3	30.5	11S 377175E 4061080N
Lake South America junction	11,040'	3.7	194.0	26.8	11S 375992E 4056208N
Shepherd Pass junction	10,910 '	0.3	194.3	26.5	11S 376045E 4055781N
Bighorn Plateau	11,430'	1.7	196.0	24.8	11S 376685E 4053326N
Wright Creek crossing	10,680'	1.9	197.9	22.9	11S 377085E 4050965N
High Sierra Trail junction	10,410'	0.8	198.7	22.1	11S 377431E 4050541N
ridge west of Mt. Young	10,960'	1.6	200.3	20.5	11S 377126E 4048918N
PCT junction west of Crabtree Meadows	10,770'	1.8	202.1	18.7	11S 378213E 4046605N
Crabtree Meadows and Crabtree Ranger Station	10,700'	0.8	202.9	17.9	11S 379241E 4047243N
Arctic Lake outlet creek crossing (Guitar Lake)	11,470 '	2.9	205.8	15.0	11S 382513E 4048029N
Mt. Whitney Trail junction	13,460'	2.6	208.4	12.4	11S 384376E 4046713N
Mt. Whitney summit	14,505'	2.0	210.4	10.4	11S 384473E 4048700N
Trail Crest	13,670'	2.1	212.5	8.3	11S 384493E 4046577N

Section 13.

Trail Crest to Whitney Portal:
Owens River (8.3 miles)

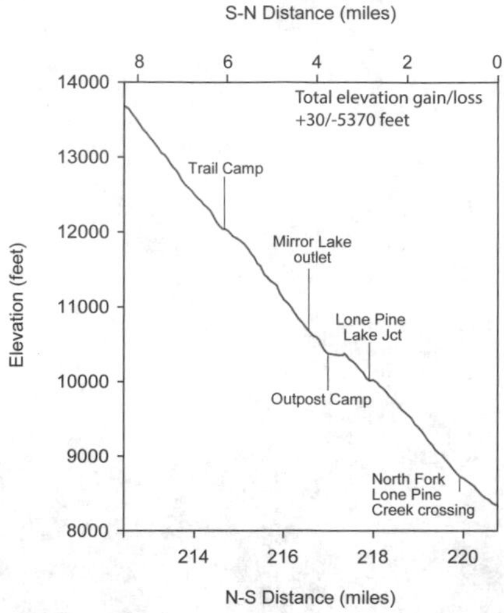

S-N Distance (miles)

Elevation (feet)

Total elevation gain/loss
+30/-5370 feet

Trail Camp

Mirror Lake
outlet

Lone Pine
Lake Jct

Outpost Camp

North Fork
Lone Pine
Creek crossing

N-S Distance (miles)

LOCATION	ELEVATION	DISTANCE FROM PREVIOUS POINT	N-S	S-N	UTM COORDINATES
Trail Crest	13,670'	—	212.5	8.3	11S 384493E 4046577N
Trail Camp	12,040'	2.2	214.7	6.1	11S 385616E 4046956N
Mirror Lake outlet	10,670'	1.9	216.6	4.2	11S 387181E 4047813N
Outpost Camp	10,370'	0.4	217.0	3.8	11S 387445E 4047888N
Lone Pine Lake junction	10,010'	0.9	217.9	2.9	11S 388197E 4048255N
North Fork Lone Pine Creek crossing	8,720'	2.1	220.0	0.8	11S 388672E 4049562N
Whitney Portal	8,330'	0.8	220.8	0.0	11S 389136E 4049566N

PANORAMAS

Panorama south from Donohue Pass

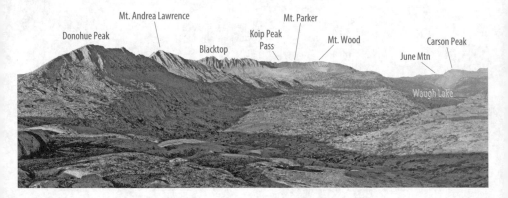

Mt. Andrea Lawrence

Mt. Parker

Donohue Peak

Koip Peak Pass

Mt. Wood

Carson Peak

Blacktop

June Mtn

Waugh Lake

Panorama north from Silver Pass; photographed by Nick Knight

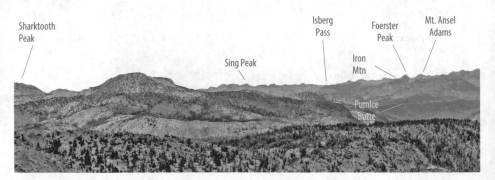

Sharktooth Peak

Isberg Pass

Foerster Peak

Mt. Ansel Adams

Sing Peak

Iron Mtn

Pumice Butte

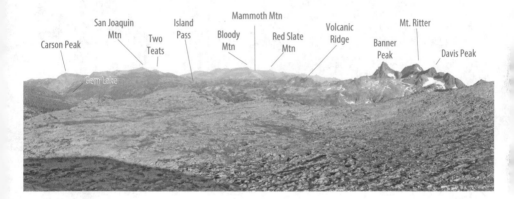

Carson Peak · Gem Lake · San Joaquin Mtn · Two Teats · Island Pass · Bloody Mtn · Mammoth Mtn · Red Slate Mtn · Volcanic Ridge · Banner Peak · Mt. Ritter · Davis Peak

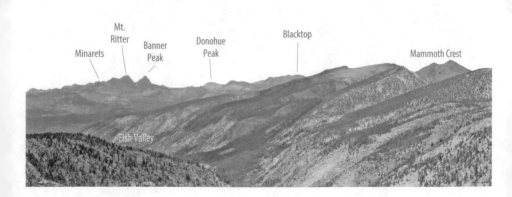

Minarets · Mt. Ritter · Banner Peak · Fish Valley · Donohue Peak · Blacktop · Mammoth Crest

Panorama north from Selden Pass

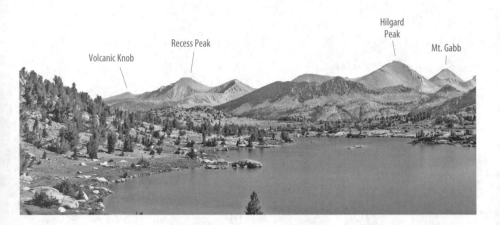

Panorama east from Muir Pass

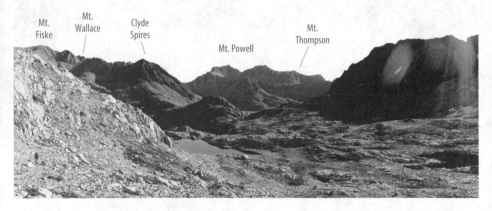

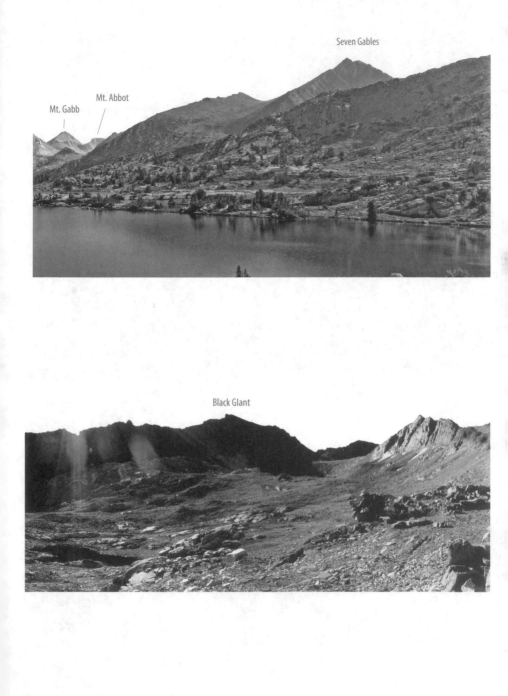

Panorama north from Mather Pass

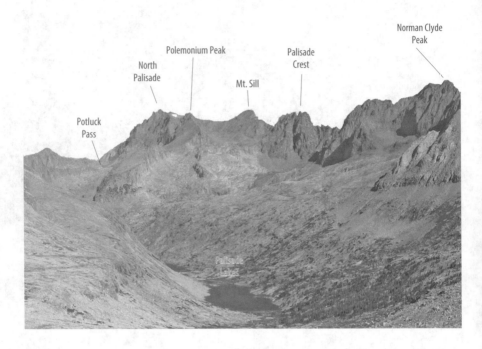

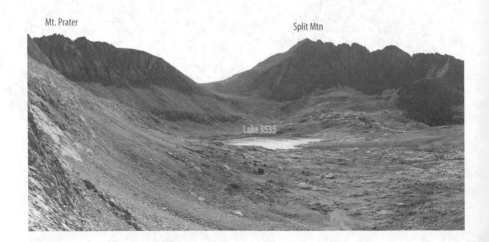

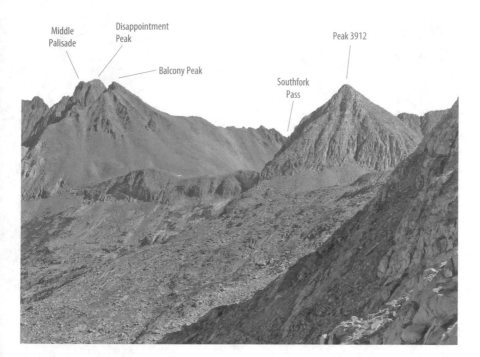

Middle Palisade

Disappointment Peak

Balcony Peak

Peak 3912

Southfork Pass

Panorama south from Mather Pass

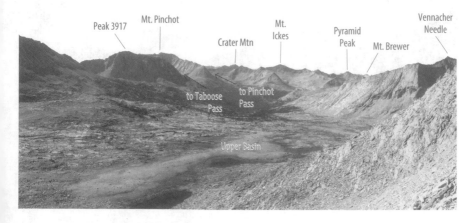

Peak 3917

Mt. Pinchot

Crater Mtn

Mt. Ickes

Pyramid Peak

Mt. Brewer

Vennacher Needle

to Taboose Pass

to Pinchot Pass

Upper Basin

Panorama north from Pinchot Pass

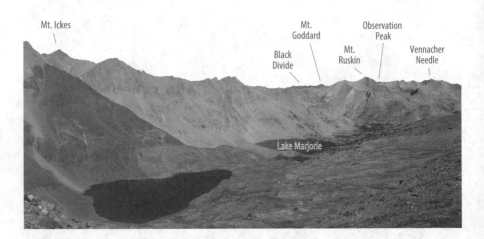

Panorama south from Pinchot Pass

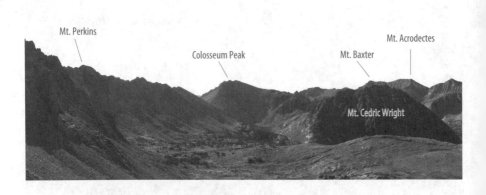

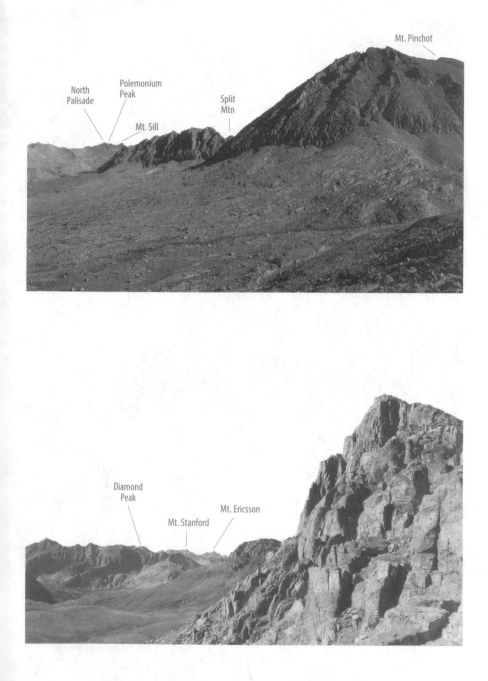

Panorama north from Glen Pass

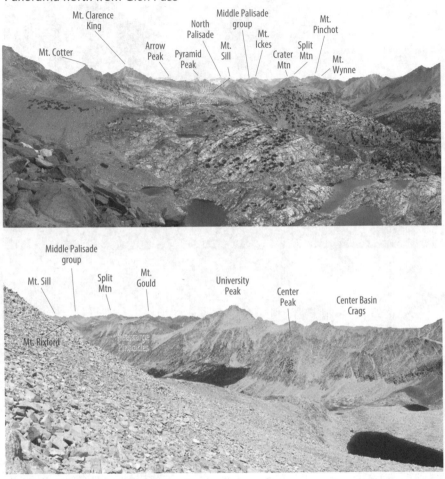

Panorama south from Forester Pass; photographed by Brad Marston

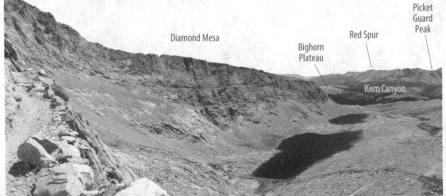

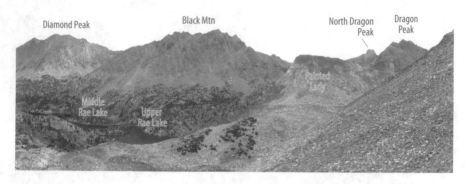

Panorama north from Forester Pass; photographed by Brad Marston

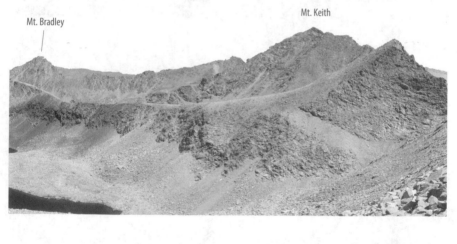

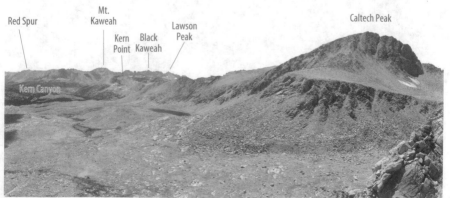

Panorama southeast from Mt. Whitney

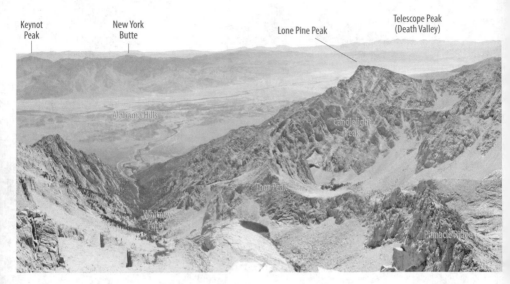

Panorama southwest from Mt. Whitney

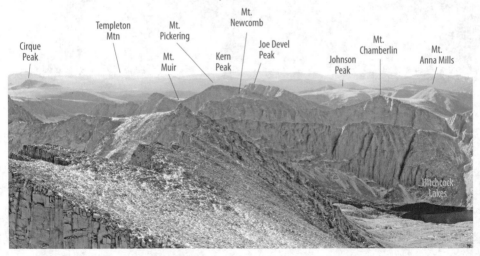

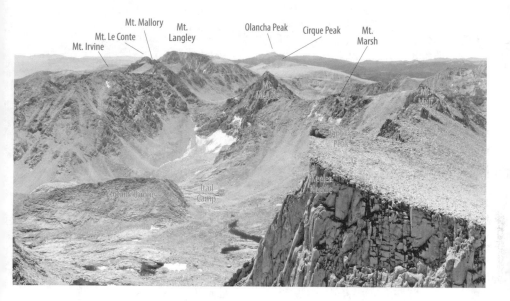

Mt. Irvine
Mt. Le Conte
Mt. Mallory
Mt. Langley
Olancha Peak
Cirque Peak
Mt. Marsh
Mt. Mallie
Mt. Muir
Cooks Peak
Keeler Needle
Wotans Throne
Trail Camp

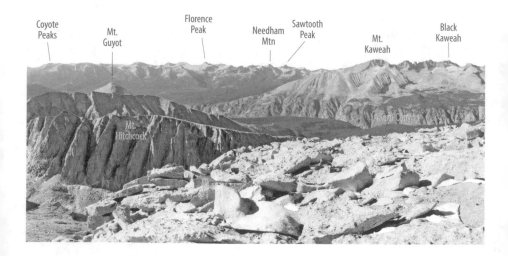

Coyote Peaks
Mt. Guyot
Florence Peak
Needham Mtn
Sawtooth Peak
Mt. Kaweah
Black Kaweah
Mt. Hitchcock
Kern Canyon

Panorama northwest from Mt. Whitney

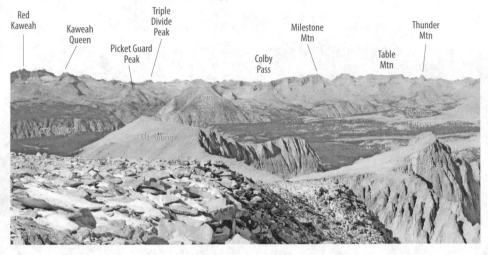

Panorama northeast from Mt. Whitney

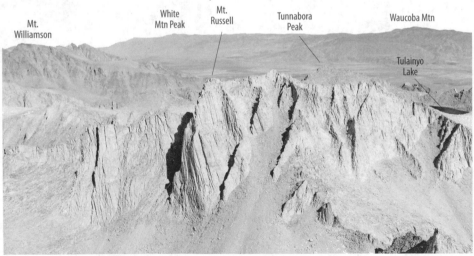

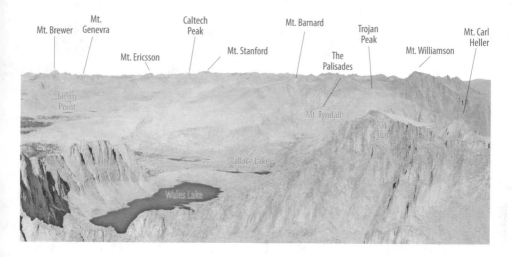

Mt. Brewer Mt. Genevra Mt. Ericsson Caltech Peak Mt. Stanford Mt. Barnard The Palisades Trojan Peak Mt. Williamson Mt. Carl Heller

Tawny Point   Mt. Tyndall   Peak 4290   Wallace Lake   Wales Lake

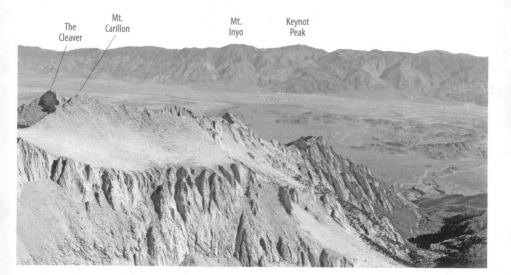

The Cleaver Mt. Carillon Mt. Inyo Keynot Peak

Owens Valley

CAMPSITES

The following table provides a selection of campsites along the JMT. It is not comprehensive, but it includes most campsites that are visible from the trail. Lacking fire rings, campsites above treeline tend to be smaller and more hidden; a few are included here, but the selection of high-elevation campsites is more sparing because many cannot sustain daily use, as would occur if they were listed here; more choices are available with a little searching. Remember that these are the coordinates where you leave the trail, not where you camp. You must be 100 feet from trail and water to camp (or 25 feet for established campsites in Kings Canyon and Sequoia National Parks). UTM coordinates indicate the location to leave the trail. If a campsite is significantly off the trail, the actual campsite location is given in parentheses. A disclaimer: UTM coordinates may be off by as much as 50 feet (15 meters), especially in deep canyons or forested areas. And remember that your GPS may also be off a little.

CAMP ID	N-S	S-N	ELEVATION	UTM COORDINATES (NAD 27)	DESCRIPTION
1.01	4.5	216.3	6,130'	11S 278399E 4179019N	large camping area in eastern Little Yosemite Valley; toilet, food-storage boxes
1.02	6.3	214.5	7,140'	11S 279291E 4180145N	many small sites to south of trail in white fir and Jeffrey pine forest
1.03	6.5	214.3	7,160'	11S 279437E 4180164N	many small sites to south of trail in white fir and Jeffrey pine forest; also small sites on the knob to the northwest of the Clouds Rest Trail junction
1.04	6.6	214.2	7,200'	11S 279547E 4180132N	large camping area by Sunrise Creek; head south from the JMT along a use trail

CAMP ID	N-S	S-N	ELEVATION	UTM COORDINATES (NAD 27)	DESCRIPTION
1.05	6.7	214.1	7,250'	11S 279655E 4180205N	site for several tents on knob with open Jeffrey pine cover and excellent views to Half Dome; head west from trail
1.06	7.1	213.7	7,430'	11S 280215E 4180266N (11S 280236E 4180229N)	large opening in Jeffrey pine/white fir forest to the south of the trail
1.07	7.2	213.6	7,470'	11S 280326E 4180338N (11S 280277E 4180367N)	head up use trail to the north; sites with excellent vistas to the west and more sheltered sites in Jeffrey pine/white fir forest to the east
1.08	8.0	212.8	7,800'	11S 281372E 4180917N	site for several tents on a little knob with Jeffrey pines above side creek; east of trail
1.09	8.1	212.7	7,830'	11S 281348E 4181052N	large opening west of creek in white fir forest; nice site
1.10	10.2	210.6	8,500'	11S 283997E 4182176N	large opening in fir forest next to a side creek; may need to detour to Sunrise Creek for water during late season
1.11	10.4	210.4	8,550'	11S 284011E 4182434N	large opening in dense fir forest alongside Sunrise Creek; head west of the trail; additional sites farther upstream to the east of the trail
1.12 Ⓧ	11.7	209.1	9,710'	11S 284852E 4183800N	large, flat, sandy site to the southeast of the trail; beautiful views but no water
1.13 Ⓧ	11.9	208.9	9,600'	11S 285079E 4184075N	site for 3–4 tents beneath open lodgepole pines at the edge of a large meadow; head south of the trail; uncertain late-season water
1.14 Ⓧ	12.1	208.7	9,580'	11S 285361E 4184157N	site for 3–4 tents beneath open lodgepole pines at the edge of a large meadow; head south of the trail; uncertain late-season water
1.15 Ⓧ	12.2	208.6	9,600'	11S 285538E 4184288N	large, flat, sandy site to the southeast of the trail; beautiful views but no water
1.16	12.8	208.0	9,320'	11S 285633E 4184995N	site for 1 tent beneath hemlocks and lodgepole pines to the northeast of the trail and creek; excellent views
1.17	13.2	207.6	9,310'	11S 285842E 4185489N (11S 285759E 4185557N)	Sunrise High Sierra Camp camping area; large area with many tent sites, a water tap, and toilet; head a short distance along the trail toward Sunrise Lakes to reach this point
1.18 Ⓧ	16.8	204.0	9,610'	11S 287693E 4190281N	openings in lodgepole pine forest and sandy flats along the southern side of Upper Cathedral Lake; do not camp in the meadow
1.19 Ⓧ	17.2	203.6	9,610'	11S 287733E 4190733N	openings in lodgepole pine forest and sandy flats along the northwest side of Upper Cathedral Lake

Ⓧ = no fires allowed

CAMP ID	N-S	S-N	ELEVATION	UTM COORDINATES (NAD 27)	DESCRIPTION
1.20 ⊗	17.7	203.1	9,430'	11S 287620E 4191522N (11S 286783E 4191387N)	many picturesque sites along the northern shore of Lower Cathedral Lake, 0.5 mile down the side trail
2.01	22.8	198.0	8,590'	11S 293123E 4194590N (11S 293077E 4194157N)	Tuolumne Meadows backpacker's campground; food-storage boxes, water, and toilets; $5 per person
2.02	28.2	192.6	8,840'	11S 298951E 4190552N	avalanche zone that marks beginning of legal camping in Lyell Canyon; hunt for options to the west of the trail, but there is no camping in the meadow
2.03	29.0	191.8	8,860'	11S 299293E 4189384N	large area under open lodgepole pine cover west of the trail
2.04	29.4	191.4	8,890'	11S 299483E 4188822N	very large area to the northwest of the Evelyn Lake junction in lodgepole pine forest
2.05	29.8	191.0	8,910'	11S 299725E 4188229N	site for 4 tents in shaded location to east of trail (toward river)
2.06	30.6	190.2	8,930'	11S 300362E 4187209N (11S 300371E 4187162N)	space for 3 tents on knob to the south of the trail
2.07	31.8	189.0	8,990'	11S 300897E 4185489N	large opening in lodgepole pine forest to the west of trail; additional smaller sites nearby; views to Mt. Lyell and Mt. Maclure from adjacent meadow
2.08	32.1	188.7	8,990'	11S 300842E 4185065N	site for 1 tent under lodgepole pine cover to the west of trail
2.09	32.4	188.4	9,070'	11S 300838E 4184616N	large area on flat shelf to the north of the trail; continue well over 100' from the trail for the best sites
2.10 ⊗	33.3	187.5	9,700'	11S 300787E 4183634N	sites for several tents on shelf above river among hemlocks and lodgepole pines; head northeast from the trail; this site is well northwest of the bridge crossing; absolutely no fires!
2.11 ⊗	33.4	187.4	9,670'	11S 300827E 4183479N	large shaded flat as one descends toward the Lyell Fork bridge; absolutely no fires!
2.12 ⊗	33.5	187.3	9,650'	11S 300871E 4183356N	2 spur trails head northeast from the southeastern side of the Lyell Fork bridge; both lead to large campsites; absolutely no fires!
2.13 ⊗	34.4	186.4	10,190'	11S 301332E 4182281N	sites for many tents beneath stunted whitebark pines to the east and northeast of the trail
2.14 ⊗	35.0	185.8	10,540'	11S 301123E 4181581N	head south from the trail to find scattered small sandy patches among slabs
3.01 ⊗	37.6	183.2	10,380'	11S 303573E 4181491N	1 well-used sandy site about 300' north of the trail; other options if you poke around; beautiful landscape of meadows and scattered whitebark pines
3.02 ⊗	38.4	182.4	10,150'	11S 304201E 4180740N	several sandy spots among slabs with scattered trees

CAMP ID	N-S	S-N	ELEVATION	UTM COORDINATES (NAD 27)	DESCRIPTION
3.03 🚫	38.7	182.1	10,070'	11S 304464E 4180314N	several sandy spots among slabs with scattered trees
3.04 🚫	38.8	182.0	10,060'	11S 304492E 4180208N	site for 4 tents under lodgepole pines a little north of the Rush Creek crossing at the Marie Lakes junction
3.05 🚫	39.7	181.1	9,680'	11S 305016E 4179603N	1 tent site in forest opening
3.06 🚫	39.9	180.9	9,630'	11S 305186E 4179516N	small site between 2 creek crossings
3.07 🚫	40.9	179.9	10,120'	11S 306395E 4179023N	single tent site under tall lodgepole pines to north of trail
4.01 🚫	41.5	179.3	10,220'	11S 306875E 4178422N	many small tent sites to either side of the trail, mostly near clusters of trees or occasionally in open z sandy flats
4.02 🚫	43.0	177.8	9,830'	11S 308733E 4177711N	head west along the use trail around Thousand Island Lake's north shore to find sandy patches among granite slabs; camping prohibited within 0.25 mile of outlet
4.03 🚫	43.2	177.6	9,820'	11S 308911E 4177556N	head west along the use trail along Thousand Island Lake's south shore; hunt for open sandy sites once past the first peninsula (camping is prohibited within 0.25 mile of the lake's outlet)
4.04 🚫	43.5	177.3	9,900'	11S 309171E 4177272N	1–2 tent sites at the edge of a small meadow southwest of the trail (above Emerald Lake)
4.05 🚫	43.8	177.0	9,940'	11S 309552E 4177027N	1 tent site on a shelf at the north end of Ruby Lake; head west from the trail
4.06 🚫	43.9	176.9	9,920'	11S 309753E 4176911N	a few small sites under hemlock trees to the southeast of Ruby Lake's outlet
4.07 🚫	45.1	175.7	9,730'	11S 310198E 4176013N	large area that can accommodate multiple parties between the trail and Garnet Lake; continue farther west around the lake for more options, looking both in forested areas and on sandy flats
4.08 🚫	45.6	175.2	9,700'	11S 310421E 4175818N	small sites along the southern shore of Garnet Lake near the island (which marks the first legal camping since the northern shore)
4.09 🚫	45.8	175.0	9,770'	11S 310343E 4175653N	sites for 2 tents in a small grove of hemlocks to the east of the trail; also sites below the trail and even more options if you descend to the lakeshore
4.10 🚫	46.3	174.5	10,110'	11S 310498E 4175326N	1 quite small site on the top of bluffs
4.11 🚫	47.9	172.9	9,190'	11S 310678E 4173859N	large open sites under a mixture of lodgepole pines, western white pines, and hemlocks to the edge of the creek (west of the trail); uncertain late-season water

🚫 = no fires allowed

CAMP ID	N-S	S-N	ELEVATION	UTM COORDINATES (NAD 27)	DESCRIPTION
4.12 Ⓧ	48.2	172.6	9,100'	11S 310869E 4173637N	large open sites under a mixture of lodgepole pines, western white pines, and hemlocks to the edge of the creek (west of the trail); surrounded by small granite outcrops; uncertain late-season water
4.13 Ⓧ	48.4	172.4	8,990'	11S 311102E 4173450N	a big open site on a bluff above the river; to the north of the trail just east of the Ediza Lake junction
4.14	50.5	170.3	9,400'	11S 312738E 4173192N	site for 1–2 tents close to Rosalie Lake's shore; descend to lake on a steep use trail
4.15	50.7	170.1	9,360'	11S 313032E 4173116N	several sites shaded by hemlocks to the southeast of Rosalie Lake's outlet; additional options 150' farther south along the trail (all campsites east of the trail)
4.16	51.3	169.5	9,580'	11S 313166E 4172571N	small site under lodgepole pines along Gladys Lake's north shore; head east from the trail
4.17	52.4	168.4	9,410'	11S 313718E 4171487N	large sandy sites to the west of the trail; this entire area was decimated by the 2011 windstorm
4.18	52.7	168.1	9,300'	11S 313999E 4171135N	flat knob with lodgepole pines that lies between the trail and the lake; head east from the trail
4.19	55.9	164.9	8,100'	11S 315137E 4167957N	small site in open lodgepole pine forest to the north of the Minaret Creek crossing; beautiful cobbled creek
4.20	56.8	164.0	7,680'	11S 315738E 4166946N (11S 316059E 4166825N)	head south and then east from the northern Devils Postpile junction to the Devils Postpile first-come, first-serve campground; do not expect to find a spot late in the day on weekends; $14 per campsite
4.21 (southbound)	59.2	161.6	7,640'	11S 316792E 4164496N (11S 316980E 4165434N)	head north from the Rainbow Falls junction to the Red's Meadow Resort and then onto the campground; follow the well-traveled trail just to the northeast of the resort area; $20 per campsite with campsites A, B, and C reserved for backpackers (also $20)
4.21 (northbound)	59.3	161.5	7,710'	11S 316898E 4164358N (11S 316980E 4165434N)	head north from the Reds Meadow junction to the Red's Meadow Resort and then onto the campground; follow the well-traveled trail just to the northeast of the resort area
4.22	62.0	158.8	8,650'	11S 318340E 4162258N	a few small sites along the southwestern slope of the northern Red Cone; head northeast from the Mammoth Pass junction
4.23	62.1	158.7	8,650'	11S 318360E 4162214N	several small sites in forest openings to the southwest of the Crater Creek crossing; area affected by blowdown, making location less appealing than before

Ⓧ = no fires allowed

CAMP ID	N-S	S-N	ELEVATION	UTM COORDINATES (NAD 27)	DESCRIPTION
5.01	65.0	155.8	9,100'	11S 320417E 4159162N	large sites that can hold many tents on the north side of Deer Creek; to the west of the trail; additional sites on the south side of Deer Creek
5.02 ⊗	70.1	150.7	9,980'	11S 325790E 4156238N	head downslope (south) from the trail to find small sites under lodgepole pines near the riverbank; parallel creek downstream to find several choices
5.03 ⊗	70.2	150.6	10,010'	11S 325837E 4156284N	2–3 small tent sites under lodgepole pines; head east toward the river; beautiful views to the Silver Divide
5.04 ⊗	70.3	150.5	10,020'	11S 325988E 4156299N	1 small site in trees south of the trail; site not visible from the trail
5.05 ⊗	72.6	148.2	9,970'	11S 327752E 4155143N	small site just near the use trail around the west side of Purple Lake; additional sites farther along the edge of Purple Lake, but fewer than previously due to 2011 blowdown
5.06 ⊗	74.4	146.4	10,390'	11S 328897E 4153694N	1 site for 3–4 tents and several smaller sites among whitebark pines on a long, low ridge to the north of the trail
5.07 ⊗	74.6	146.2	10,340'	11S 329090E 4153664N	several small sites among whitebark pines on slight knobs to the south of the trail
5.08 ⊗	76.9	143.9	9,510'	11S 329800E 4151887N	site for 2 small tents between the trail and Fish Creek
5.09 ⊗	77.0	143.8	9,490'	11S 329681E 4151743N	medium-size sloping site in open lodgepole pine forest along a stretch of Cascade Creek with big pools and slabs; north of (above) the trail
5.10 ⊗	77.7	143.1	9,210'	11S 329249E 4151040N	site for 3 tents in hemlock and fir forest, bit south of Fish Creek bridge; head west of the trail
5.11 ⊗	77.8	143.0	9,200'	11S 329201E 4150946N	site for 2 tents on open sandy knob just north of Cascade Valley (Fish Creek) junction; head west of the trail
5.12 ⊗	78.4	142.4	9,500'	11S 329052E 4150512N	small sites among heath vegetation and hemlocks on a small bench; west of the trail; water in gully below
5.13 ⊗	78.4	142.4	9,510'	11S 328997E 4150443N	2 tiny sites among heath vegetation and hemlocks on a small bench; west of the trail; water in gully below
5.14 ⊗	78.9	141.9	9,740'	11S 329012E 4149830N	several big sites beneath scattered lodgepole pines to edge of small marsh; south of trail
5.15 ⊗	79.1	141.7	9,860'	11S 329191E 4149663N	1–2 tent sites beneath scattered lodgepole pines; to south of trail
5.16 ⊗	80.0	140.8	10,290'	11S 329931E 4149425N	small sandy sites among slabs, mostly on the northeast side of Squaw Lake outlet; open views and evening sun

CAMP ID	N-S	S-N	ELEVATION	UTM COORDINATES (NAD 27)	DESCRIPTION
5.17 ⊗	80.6	140.2	10,540'	11S 329563E 4148911N	walk 100' from the trail (and water) and search for sandy spots that hold a single tent; the options are not visible from the trail
6.01 ⊗	82.4	138.4	10,440'	11S 330404E 4147228N	small sandy sites beneath pines scattered near the eastern shore of Silver Pass Lake; head west from trail
6.02	83.8	137.0	9,790'	11S 330076E 4145555N	several sites, each for 1–2 tents along Silver Pass Creek under scattered lodgepole pines; head west from trail
6.03	84.3	136.5	9,640'	11S 330724E 4145272N	several large sites, including a stock camp, across the large meadow; look on low knobs in the meadow for options; difficult to access during high water
6.04	85.2	135.6	8,990'	11S 331344E 4145016N	small site beneath forest cover near the Mott Lake junction; head west from trail
6.05	85.4	135.4	8,920'	11S 331289E 4144649N	2 tent sites under lodgepole pines between the trail and the creek; at the edge of Pocket Meadow
6.06	85.6	135.2	8,900'	11S 331220E 4144491N	space for several tents under lodgepole pines between the trail and the creek; at the southern end of Pocket Meadow where the creek is beginning to flow over slabs again
6.07	85.7	135.1	8,860'	11S 331150E 4144249N	site for a few tents on the west side of the creek under lodgepole pines; only accessible during low water
6.08	86.7	134.1	8,320'	11S 330975E 4143090N	site for 3–4 tents in open Jeffrey pine forest opening to the south of the trail
6.09	87.4	133.4	7,970'	11S 330604E 4142489N	site for 2 tents in white fir forest on the south side of Silver Pass Creek
6.10	87.4	133.4	7,960'	11S 330589E 4142519N	room for several tents in a shaded opening on the north side of Silver Pass Creek
6.11	88.1	132.7	7,880'	11S 329855E 4142137N	site for a few tents on an open flat with Jeffrey pines and junipers; head east of the trail
6.12	88.1	132.7	7,890'	11S 329825E 4142088N	big area on an open bench overlooking Mono Creek; to the west of the trail
6.13	93.5	127.3	9,300'	11S 331561E 4138309N	3 tent spots on a knob shaded by large Jeffrey pines and junipers to the south of the trail; uncertain late-season water
6.14	94.0	126.8	9,080'	11S 332005E 4137951N	2 small tent sites to the west of the trail
6.15	94.8	126.0	8,940'	11S 332846E 4137180N	large area on the north side of Bear Creek; follow the Bear Creek Trail west
6.16	95.0	125.8	8,990'	11S 333115E 4136988N	4 tent spots on slabs and sand between the trail and Bear Creek

CAMP ID	N-S	S-N	ELEVATION	UTM COORDINATES (NAD 27)	DESCRIPTION
6.17	95.3	125.5	9,090'	11S 333381E 4136567N	space for 3–4 tents in a lodgepole pine–covered flat between the trail and Bear Creek
6.18	95.4	125.4	9,080'	11S 333397E 4136452N	sites for at least 4 tents under lodgepole pines between the trail and Bear Creek
6.19	95.9	124.9	9,160'	11S 333630E 4135826N	site for 3–4 tents in a lodgepole pine–covered flat; head east from trail, away from Bear Creek
6.20	96.3	124.5	9,230'	11S 333765E 4135263N	large area under lodgepole pines between the trail and Bear Creek; tent sites dispersed and numerous
6.21	96.6	124.2	9,280'	11S 333762E 4134754N	2–3 tent sites in lodgepole pine forest between Bear Creek and trail
6.22	96.8	124.0	9,320'	11S 333918E 4134609N	site in open lodgepole pine forest just south of the Hilgard Branch
6.23	97.9	122.9	9,580'	11S 334689E 4133057N	spaces for 2 tents at the border of forest and expansive slabs; head west from trail
6.24	98.0	122.8	9,570'	11S 334645E 4132938N	several tent sites along the eastern bank of Bear Creek, south of the trail
6.25 🚫	99.0	121.8	10,020'	11S 334417E 4131831N	several sites, each for 2–3 tents on the low knob to the east of the trail
6.26 🚫	99.3	121.5	10,030'	11S 334188E 4131442N	open site for 2 tents to the east of the trail; also a large site a short distance along the Rose Lake Trail
6.27 🚫	100.7	120.1	10,570'	11S 334221E 4129672N	a few small sites, always for 1–2 tents, under whitebark pines around the western shore of Marie Lake; ensure you are 100' from water
7.01 🚫	102.5	118.3	10,570'	11S 333869E 4127470N	site for 1–2 tents on open slabs near Heart Lake's outlet; head west from trail
7.02 🚫	103.2	117.6	10,220'	11S 333771E 4126784N	2 tent sites on open knob east of Upper Sallie Keyes Lake; head west from trail
7.03 🚫	103.4	117.4	10,190'	11S 333812E 4126598N	large area in lodgepole pine forest between the 2 Sallie Keyes Lakes; head west from trail
7.04 🚫	103.6	117.2	10,190'	11S 333726E 4126332N	sites for many tents in lodgepole pine forest to the north of the outlet of Sallie Keyes Lakes
7.05 🚫	104.5	116.3	10,010'	11S 333867E 4125239N	large open area under scattered lodgepole pines; water in nearby meadow
7.06 🚫	104.8	116.0	10,100'	11S 334037E 4125007N	sites for 4+ tents on knob ringed by lodgepole pines with a beautiful view; water is along the trail just to the south
7.07	105.8	115.0	9,740'	11S 334706E 4124395N	small site in lodgepole pine forest along the southern bank of Senger Creek; head west from trail

🚫 = no fires allowed

CAMP ID	N-S	S-N	ELEVATION	UTM COORDINATES (NAD 27)	DESCRIPTION
7.08	107.9	111.1	7,700'	11S 334050E 4123185N or 11S 334958E 4121342N (11S 333302E 4122384N)	many sites beneath scattered trees and in sandy spots on slabs near Blayney Hot Springs; just before Muir Trail Ranch you reach a junction and head left (south) along the use trail toward the river
7.09	107.9	111.1	7,800'	11S 334050E 4123185N or 11S 334958E 4121342N (11S 334425E 4121699N)	slightly sloping bench with room for 2 tents on a shelf along the South Fork of the San Joaquin River; on southern cutoff trail to Muir Trail Ranch
7.10	107.9	111.1	7,800'	11S 334050E 4123185N or 11S 334958E 4121342N (11S 334525E 4121555N)	lodgepole pine flat with room for several tents along the South Fork of the San Joaquin River; on southern cutoff trail to Muir Trail Ranch
7.11	111.5	109.3	8,060'	11S 337471E 4121235N	site beneath open Jeffrey pines on the southeast side of the bridge at the Piute Pass junction
7.12	111.5	109.3	8,050'	11S 337507E 4121196N	large sites in sandy openings beneath junipers, Jeffrey pines, and white firs; head west from the trail
7.13	111.7	109.1	8,070'	11S 337720E 4121059N	space for 2–3 tents on lodgepole pine flat along the creek; head west from trail
7.14	111.9	108.9	8,110'	11S 337987E 4120836N	site for 3 tents on sandy shelf above the creek; head west from trail
7.15	112.9	107.9	8,230'	11S 338923E 4119903N	sandy, open spot with space for 2 tents; just west of the trail
7.16	113.0	107.8	8,250'	11S 339017E 4119840N	tiny sandy spot that holds 1 tent; just west of the trail
7.17	113.0	107.8	8,240'	11S 339105E 4119796N	room for 2 tents on a lodgepole pine–shaded shelf above the river; head west from the trail
7.18	114.1	106.7	8,390'	11S 340259E 4118713N	very large area with room for many groups in lodgepole pine forest; from the southwest side of the bridge, head north on a spur trail
7.19	114.3	106.5	8,420'	11S 340410E 4118493N	space for several tents in an open area ringed by scattered trees; just east of the trail
7.20	114.9	105.9	8,470'	11S 340709E 4117643N	big area up a small hill to the west of the trail; used as a stock camp
7.21	115.0	105.8	8,480'	11S 340786E 4117577N	space for several groups in open lodgepole pine stands along the southeastern side of the river; head south from the east side of the bridge
7.22	115.2	105.6	8,480'	11S 340783E 4117874N	large area under lodgepole pine cover just before the switchbacks to Evolution Valley begin
7.23	116.4	104.4	9,190'	11S 341729E 4117814N	small, sandy spots for 3–4 tents on a bluff above the trail; head south on a steep use trail
7.24	116.8	104.0	9,240'	11S 342109E 4117988N	small spot on bench shaded by lodgepole pines; between trail and river
7.25	116.9	103.9	9,240'	11S 342286E 4117985N	large opening ringed by lodgepole pines (stock camp); between trail and river

CAMP ID	N-S	S-N	ELEVATION	UTM COORDINATES (NAD 27)	DESCRIPTION
7.26	117.2	103.6	9,240'	11S 342682E 4117873N	sites for 3 tents in opening between the trail and Evolution Meadow
7.27	117.3	103.5	9,240'	11S 343886E 4117336N	small site beneath scattered lodgepole pines; to the north of the trail
7.28	118.1	102.7	9,470'	11S 344611E 4117057N	2–3 tent sites on sandy shelf; between trail and river
7.29	118.7	102.1	9,540'	11S 345069E 4116998N	open lodgepole pine flat at the western edge of McClure Meadow; between trail and river
7.30	119.0	101.8	9,630'	11S 345128E 4116984N	several medium-size sites at the western end of McClure Meadow, with beautiful views to Mt. Darwin and the Hermit; additional sites 100–200' farther east along trail
7.31	119.3	101.5	9,650'	11S 345497E 4116932N	several small- to large-size sites toward the eastern end of McClure Meadow, with beautiful views to Mt. Darwin and the Hermit
7.32	119.7	101.1	9,680'	11S 346123E 4116652N	2–3 tent sites in opening in lodgepole pine forest; stretch of river with pools and small cascades
7.33	120.0	100.8	9,740'	11S 346431E 4116516N	large site in a lodgepole pine flat; between the trail and river
7.34	121.4	99.4	9,940'	11S 347937E 4115348N	site for 2–3 tents on open slabs just south of the Darwin Bench drainage; views to the Hermit; between trail and river
7.35 🚫	122.9	97.9	10,830'	11S 348924E 4115318N	space for 1–2 tents among whitebark pines at a tarn below Evolution Lake; head downslope (east) from the trail
7.36 🚫	123.1	97.7	10,860'	11S 349130E 4115124N	sandy site for 1–2 tents among slabs to the south of the trail; make sure you use a previously used site
7.37 🚫	125.1	95.7	10,980'	11S 349525E 4112936N	many options along the eastern shore of Sapphire Lake; cross the lake's outlet and walk along the eastern shore, ensuring you are 100' from water and not camped on any plants
7.38 🚫	127.0	93.8	11,430'	11S 349306E 4110304N	space for ~5 small tents, distributed over a large area near the Wanda Lake outlet; each site is small, sandy, and surrounded by slabs; beautiful views
7.39 🚫	127.7	93.1	11,460'	11S 350097E 4109536N	space for 2 tents on the shallow ridge that separates the trail from Wanda Lake; lovely views of Evolution Basin
8.01 🚫	129.6	91.2	11,690'	11S 352132E 4108629N (11S 352105E 4108700N)	sandy site for 1–2 tents among slabs next to a small tarn above Helen Lake; head 200' northwest from the trail
8.02 🚫	131.2	89.6	11,150'	11S 353543E 4109680N	space for 1 tent in a sandy patch on a whitebark pine–covered knob
8.03 🚫	132.0	88.8	10,840'	11S 354190E 4109551N	2 sandy tent sites at the southeastern edge of Lake 10,800+; excellent views

🚫 = no fires allowed

CAMP ID	N-S	S-N	ELEVATION	UTM COORDINATES (NAD 27)	DESCRIPTION
8.04 ⊗	132.0	88.8	10,850'	11S 354255E 4109426N	big site on shelf to the east of the creek
8.05 ⊗	132.3	88.5	10,700'	11S 354266E 4109185N	2 tent sites in small opening beneath whitebark pines; head east from the trail
8.06 ⊗	132.4	88.4	10,640'	11S 354389E 4109048N	1 tent site under lodgepole pines to the west of the trail; good views to the Black Giant
8.07 ⊗	132.7	88.1	10,470'	11S 354408E 4108809N	lodgepole pine flat above river with space for quite a few tents; good views to the Black Giant; head west from trail
8.08 ⊗	133.0	87.8	10,320'	11S 354628E 4108612N	Starrs Camp; at least 5 tent sites among young lodgepole pines to the south of the trail; beautiful views of Langille Peak, the Black Giant, and Le Conte Canyon
8.09	134.2	86.6	9,480'	11S 356026E 4108399N	sites for 5 tents beside creek just south of the switchbacks
8.10	134.5	86.3	9,380'	11S 356447E 4108399N	2–3 tent sites on sandy bench above river
8.11	134.8	86.0	9,310'	11S 356939E 4108489N	large area under lodgepole pine cover between the trail and river
8.12	135.2	85.6	9,250'	11S 357367E 4108394N	space for many tents (across several small sites) in openings in lodgepole pine forest; just south of Big Pete Creek crossing
8.13	135.4	85.4	9,230'	11S 357585E 4108192N	Big Pete Meadow; lateral trail to large site by creek under lodgepole pine cover
8.14	135.8	85.0	9,010'	11S 357827E 4107654N	space for 1–2 tents on a sandy shelf with excellent views of Langille Peak and to the south; head west from trail
8.15	136.1	84.7	8,860'	11S 357968E 4107320N	site for 2 tents under lodgepole pines; head west from trail
8.16	136.2	84.6	8,860'	11S 358043E 4107208N	Little Pete Meadow; big stock camp under lodgepole pine cover at edge of meadow; head west from trail
8.17	136.9	83.9	8,740'	11S 358394E 4106307N (11S 358437E 4106267N)	2 sites in sandy flats among slabs with good views; walk a short distance up the Bishop Pass Trail (to coordinates) and then head south
8.18	136.9	83.9	8,720'	11S 358405E 4106254N	big areas under lodgepole pines; head west from trail
8.19	137.0	83.8	8,710'	11S 358413E 4106202N	space for 5 tents under lodgepole pines; head west from trail; additional site closer to the Dusy Fork bridge
8.20	137.1	83.7	8,690'	11S 358390E 4105977N	spot for 1–2 tents under lodgepole pines; head east from trail
8.21	137.3	83.5	8,640'	11S 358282E 4105738N	spot for 1–2 tents under lodgepole pines; head west from trail
8.22	137.4	83.4	8,640'	11S 358319E 4105633N	site for 2–3 tents under lodgepole pines with views to the Citadel; head west from trail
8.23	138.3	82.5	8,350'	11S 358159E 4104265N	space for 3 tents on open bench above river; head west from trail

CAMP ID	N-S	S-N	ELEVATION	UTM COORDINATES (NAD 27)	DESCRIPTION
8.24	139.3	81.5	8,240'	11S 358792E 4102912N	space for 5 tents at the edge of Grouse Meadow; head west from trail
8.25	139.3	81.5	8,250'	11S 358854E 4102835N	space for 3 tents at the edge of Grouse Meadow; head west from trail
8.26	139.4	81.4	8,240'	11S 358908E 4102796N	site for 1 tent under lodgepole pines near the edge of Grouse Meadow; head east from trail
8.27	140.3	80.5	8,050'	11S 359614E 4101718N	several large sites beneath Jeffrey pines at the Middle Fork Trail junction; head south from trail
8.28	141.4	79.4	8,430'	11S 361063E 4101688N	2 tent sites on shelf above creek with some lodgepole pine cover; head south from trail
8.29	141.6	79.2	8,430'	11S 361299E 4101671N	2 small tent sites under Jeffrey pines; head north from trail
8.30	143.0	77.8	8,680'	11S 363369E 4101721N	site for 4+ tents on lodgepole pine flat between trail and river; pocket of trees within the burn area
8.31	143.3	77.5	8,730'	11S 363705E 4101859N	space for 4 tents in lodgepole pine flat between trail and river; pocket of trees within the burn area
8.32	143.8	77.0	8,870'	11S 364434E 4101985N	Deer Meadow; very large site beneath lodgepole pine forest just east of creek crossing draining Palisade Basin; head south from trail
8.33	144.3	76.5	8,890'	11S 365009E 4101799N	large areas under lodgepole pines and big red firs near the base of the Golden Staircase; head south from trail
8.34	144.4	76.4	8,960'	11S 365252E 4101832N	2–3 tent sites under lodgepole pines and red firs near the base of the Golden Staircase; head south from trail
8.35 ⊗	146.5	74.3	10,360'	11S 367067E 4101836N	space for 1–2 tents on sandy flat next to hemlocks; head southeast from trail; good views to west
8.36 ⊗	147.2	73.6	10,590'	11S 367592E 4102422N	2 tent spots in sandy patches between slabs; head south from trail
8.37 ⊗	147.3	73.5	10,600'	11S 367773E 4102386N	Lower Palisade Lake; lots of small sandy spots among slabs, both north of lake and southwest of lake at outlet; views to the Middle Palisade group
8.38 ⊗	148.2	72.6	10,790'	11S 368796E 4101960N	2 sandy sites under whitebark pines; head south from trail; additional options southeast along the trail
8.39 ⊗	148.4	72.4	10,840'	11S 369099E 4101740N	many sites near each other; all sandy spots among slabs, surrounded by whitebark pines and overlooking Upper Palisade Lake; excellent views; water a short distance south on trail

⊗ = no fires allowed

CAMP ID		N–S	S–N	ELEVATION	UTM COORDINATES (NAD 27)	DESCRIPTION
8.40	(X)	148.5	72.3	10,840'	11S 369143E 4101671N	several sandy sites with whitebark pines on the northwest side of the creek
8.41	(X)	148.6	72.2	10,850'	11S 369251E 4101490N	space for 3 tents beneath stunted whitebark pines and overlooking Upper Palisade Lake; excellent views; head west of trail
8.42	(X)	149.1	71.7	10,970'	11S 369524E 4100850N	1–2 small tent sites under last white-bark pines; amazing views down to the Palisade Lakes
9.01	(X)	152.1	68.7	11,610'	11S 370721E 4098884N	Upper Basin; head due east to reach large lake with many flat, sandy tent sites; beautiful surroundings
9.02	(X)	152.5	68.3	11,500'	11S 370468E 4098259N	wander in any direction to find sandy tent sites near the many tarns in Upper Basin; make sure you camp on unvegetated areas 100' from water
9.03		155.3	65.5	10,570'	11S 371168E 4094326N	search around for options toward stream; east of the trail
9.04	(X)	156.3	64.5	10,190'	11S 371685E 4092851N	site for 5 tents in open flat just east of trail
9.05	(X)	156.3	64.5	10,170'	11S 371672E 4092792N	from cairn marking abandoned Taboose Pass Trail, head east to creek; here there is a large opening under lodgepole pines
9.06	(X)	156.7	64.1	10,050'	11S 371502E 4092346N	several sites for 1–2 tents in lodge-pole pine forest on the south side of the river crossing; head east from trail
9.07	(X)	156.7	64.1	10,050'	11S 371517E 4092288N	several tent sites in sandy openings to the west of the trail; farther from water than previous camp
9.08	(X)	158.1	62.7	10,860'	11S 372161E 4091060N	2–3 small tent sites just next to trail; some to the east and others to the west
9.09	(X)	158.4	62.4	11,000'	11S 372292E 4090590N	tent sites on small knob with white-bark pines; head west toward a tarn
9.10	(X)	158.7	62.1	11,050'	11S 372478E 4090187N	5+ individual tent sites in sandy spots among slabs and whitebark pines between two small lakes
9.11	(X)	158.9	61.9	11,080'	11S 372495E 4090007N	sandy site for 1 tent near the lake; head west of trail
9.12	(X)	159.1	61.7	11,130'	11S 372595E 4089730N	1–2 tent sites in sandy location near the north shore of Lake Marjorie
9.13	(X)	159.2	61.6	11,150'	11S 372766E 4089702N	a few sandy spots on either side of the trail; landscape of slabs and whitebark pines
9.14	(X)	159.5	61.3	11,250'	11S 373005E 4089464N	2 small sites among whitebark pines; head east from trail; water a short walk up the trail
9.15	(X)	159.7	61.1	11,280'	11S 373120E 4089338N	1–2 sandy spots on slab west of the trail; water a short walk down the trail
9.16	(X)	160.2	60.6	11,580'	11S 373640E 4088926N	big sandy flat below the trail; good late-season site but could be damp earlier; beautiful views

CAMP ID	N-S	S-N	ELEVATION	UTM COORDINATES (NAD 27)	DESCRIPTION
10.01 🚫	162.6	58.2	11,380'	11S 375436E 4087425N	head 500' north to the chain of small lakes; hunt for sandy flats among whitebark pines, ensuring you are camped off vegetation
10.02 🚫	163.7	57.1	10,890'	11S 375735E 4086049N	big site in an opening on a knob, surrounded by lodgepole pines; head south from the trail (away from the lake)
10.03 🚫	164.2	56.6	10,610'	11S 375520E 4085427N (11S 375607E 4085397N)	head 300' east toward the outlet of Twin Lakes; space for 2 tents beneath lodgepole pines
10.04 🚫	164.7	56.1	10,350'	11S 375315E 4084786N	small site east of Sawmill Trail junction under lodgepole pine cover with wet streamside vegetation; cross to east side of creek
10.05	165.5	55.3	9,800'	11S 374383E 4084432N	big site on a shelf shaded by lodgepole pines; head east from trail
10.06	166.6	54.2	9,240'	11S 373453E 4083300N	several tent sites on bench above river partially shaded by lodgepole pines; head south from trail
10.07	168.4	52.4	8,520'	11S 371951E 4081594N	large site just south of Woods Creek crossing with room for 20 parties; additional sites on the knob to the southwest of the trail; food-storage boxes
10.08	170.8	50.0	9,450'	11S 374029E 4079218N	several small sites under lodgepole pine cover to the east of a marshy area; head south from trail
10.09 🚫	172.4	48.4	10,220'	11S 374516E 4077255N	many sites along the north shore of Dollar Lake; beautiful reflections of Fin Dome in the lake
10.10 🚫	172.4	48.4	10,220'	11S 374487E 4077241N	sites along the west shore of Dollar Lake; head east from trail, taking note of the restoration areas
10.11 🚫	173.0	47.8	10,310'	11S 374369E 4076481N	Arrowhead Lake; first tent sites are beneath lodgepole pines near where you leave the trail; continue south, paralleling the lakeshore for many more options both under forest cover and on shady knobs even farther south; fantastic view of Fin Dome; food-storage box
10.12 🚫	173.9	46.9	10,560'	11S 374721E 4075127N	large sites in sandy flats with sparse lodgepole pine cover; on bench overlooking Lower Rae Lake
10.13 🚫	174.0	46.8	10,570'	11S 374760E 4075057N	Lower Rae Lake; large sites in sandy flats with sparse lodgepole pine cover; on bench overlooking Lower Rae Lake; food-storage box
10.14 🚫	174.2	46.6	10,590'	11S 375019E 4074783N	few small sandy sites on a shelf overlooking Middle Rae Lake
10.15 🚫	174.4	46.4	10,590'	11S 375188E 4074573N	1 tent site on sandy bench above Middle Rae Lake; beautiful views to the Painted Lady

🚫 = no fires allowed

CAMP ID	N-S	S-N	ELEVATION	UTM COORDINATES (NAD 27)	DESCRIPTION
10.16 ⊗	174.8	46.0	10,610'	11S 375377E 4074106N	Middle Rae Lake; very large camping area along the shore of Middle Rae Lake; head 500' west on a spur trail toward lake; food-storage boxes
10.17 ⊗	175.4	45.4	10,560'	11S 374963E 4073711N	5 small sandy spots, each for 1 tent, among slabs and whitebark pines scattered around the Sixty Lake Basin junction; most sites are not visible from the trail; fantastic views of the Painted Lady and Upper Rae Lake
10.18 ⊗	176.2	44.6	11,090'	11S 374583E 4073136N	space for 2–3 tents in a cluster of whitebark pines on a knob with a tarn behind; head northwest from trail
10.19 ⊗	176.5	44.3	11,380'	11S 374331E 4072689N	exposed alpine sites in sandy patches between slabs by tarns to west of trail; sites best seen when you are slightly above them
11.01 ⊗	177.7	43.1	11,570'	11S 373961E 4071908N	several small sites among whitebark pines near the lake outlet; head east from trail
11.02 ⊗	179.6	41.2	10,740'	11S 373685E 4070166N (11S 372780E 4070952N)	large area in lodgepole pine forest at the north end of Charlotte Lake; food-storage box; 0.9 mile off the JMT on the trail to Charlotte Lake
11.03 ⊗	180.0	40.8	10,520'	11S 374110E 4069887N	small sites among streamside vegetation and foxtail pines at Bullfrog Lake Junction; head east from trail
11.04 ⊗	180.2	40.6	10,360'	11S 374160E 4069650N	site for a few tents on shelf above creek with lodgepole pine cover and wet heath vegetation; head south from trail
11.05 ⊗	180.6	40.2	10,070'	11S 374409E 4069459N	2–3 shaded tent sites under lodgepole pines to the west of the creek crossing; head south from trail
11.06	181.1	39.7	9,550'	11S 374054E 4069011N	large sites in wet (and often buggy) lodgepole pine forest just upstream of Bubbs Creek junction; head south from trail
11.07	181.4	39.4	9,530'	11S 374419E 4068919N	2 spots next to trail in dry lodgepole pine forest; just north of Vidette Meadow
11.08	181.5	39.3	9,540'	11S 374566E 4068865N	Vidette Meadow; several large sites in opening in dry lodgepole pine forest at edge of Vidette Meadow; views to East Vidette; food-storage box
11.09	181.6	39.2	9,550'	11S 374670E 4068796N	large site in dry lodgepole pine forest at edge of Vidette Meadow; views to East Vidette; more options 200' south
11.10	182.4	38.4	9,910'	11S 375616E 4068174N	Upper Vidette Meadow; large opening in flat lodgepole pine forest; food-storage box
11.11 ⊗	182.6	38.2	9,960'	11S 375833E 4068121N	large site in dry lodgepole pine forest; head west from trail
11.12 ⊗	184.0	36.8	10,400'	11S 376951E 4066475N	space for a few tents on a shelf between the trail and stream; under lodgepole pine cover

CAMP ID	N-S	S-N	ELEVATION	UTM COORDINATES (NAD 27)	DESCRIPTION
11.13 🚫	184.3	36.5	10,460'	11S 377220E 4066135N	2 small sites under lodgepole pines; head east from trail
11.14 🚫	184.3	36.5	10,480'	11S 377256E 4066060N	Center Basin junction; lots of sandy sites among slabs above the river and on a lodgepole pine flat; head west from trail; food-storage box
11.15 🚫	184.7	36.1	10,530'	11S 377492E 4065690N	sites for ~5 tents just to the south of the Center Basin creek crossing; look to both sides of the trail
11.16 🚫	185.6	35.2	10,910'	11S 377616E 4064562N	3–4 small tent sites on small knob with whitebark pines; seasonal trickle nearby; spectacular views; uncertain late-season water
11.17 🚫	185.6	35.2	10,930'	11S 377584E 4064455N	3–4 small tent sites on flat shelf with scattered whitebark pines above valley; seasonal trickle nearby; spectacular views; uncertain late-season water
11.18 🚫	186.1	34.7	11,230'	11S 377550E 4063727N	several single tent sites beneath last stand of foxtail pines; excellent views
11.19 🚫	186.2	34.6	11,240'	11S 377587E 4063736N	a few small spots in sandy flats, mostly without tree cover; amazing views
11.20 🚫	187.2	33.6	11,770'	11S 378141E 4063449N	2 small sandy tent sites among slabs and boulders near the small tarn to the east of the trail; be sure to keep off alpine plants
11.21 🚫	188.1	32.7	12,240'	11S 377824E 4062542N	a few exposed tent sites overlooking Lake 12,250 and surrounded by talus; excellent views to Junction Peak
12.01 🚫	190.2	30.6	12,500'	11S 377308E 4061263N	a few sandy flats among slabs near the outlet of the first lake south of Forester Pass
12.02 🚫	191.1	29.7	12,270'	11S 376837E 4060044N	2 tent sites in sandy flat; open landscape; seasonal water nearby but lakes farther away
12.03 🚫	191.2	29.6	12,220'	11S 376811E 4059934N	sandy tent site just southeast of the trail, with additional options if you continue to nearby lakes
12.04 🚫	193.2	27.6	11,360'	11S 375960E 4057330N	1 site in big grove of foxtail pines east of the trail; seeps with water nearby but uncertain late-season water
12.05 🚫	194.1	26.7	10,980'	11S 376041E 4055999N	site for 1–2 tents in sandy opening to the north of the trail
12.06 🚫	194.1	26.7	10,970'	11S 376052E 4055967N	Tyndall Creek crossing; space for 4+ tents in the large sandy opening to the west of trail; search farther west and south for other options; food-storage box
12.07 🚫	194.4	26.4	10,880'	11S 375984E 4055650N	several sandy sites just north of the Tyndall ranger cabin junction; head west from trail
12.08 🚫	194.8	26.0	11,030'	11S 376211E 4055104N	Tyndall Frog Ponds; large sites under open lodgepole pines; look on both sides of the trail; food-storage box

🚫 = no fires allowed

CAMP ID	N-S	S-N	ELEVATION	UTM COORDINATES (NAD 27)	DESCRIPTION
12.09 🐾	196.0	24.8	11,430'	11S 376685E 4053326N	lots of flat, sandy spots along the northern side of the lake on Bighorn Plateau; no trees or large rocks for shelter; make sure you camp off vegetation and 100' away from the lake
12.10 🐾	197.6	23.2	10,800'	11S 377308E 4051328N	lodgepole pine–shaded sites on shelf above Wright Creek; head south from trail
12.11 🐾	197.9	22.9	10,690'	11S 377081E 4050929N	a few sites in a lodgepole pine–shaded opening to the south of Wright Creek; head west from trail; additional options another 100' to the south
12.12 🐾	198.6	22.2	10,410'	11S 377432E 4050541N	large site near the High Sierra Trail junction, adjacent to open meadow
12.13 🐾	198.7	22.1	10,400'	11S 377464E 4050477N	Wallace Creek crossing; many sites under scattered lodgepole pines on the southwest side of Wallace Creek; continue another 100' to the south for additional choices; food-storage box
12.14 🐾	198.8	22.0	10,460'	11S 377680E 4050493N	open sandy campsite, but it is a 500' walk to Wallace Creek for water
12.15 🐾	199.2	21.6	10,650'	11S 377495E 4050180N	2 tent sites under lodgepole pines just north of a small creek; head east from trail
12.16 🐾	200.8	20.0	10,700'	11S 377402E 4048191N	2 tent sites at edge of Sandy Meadow in mixed foxtail and lodge-pole pine forest to the west of the creek crossing; head south from trail; uncertain late-season water
12.17 🐾	202.8	18.0	10,670'	11S 379142E 4047130N	large site under lodgepole pine forest to the east of trail
12.18 🐾	202.9	17.9	10,770'	11S 379241E 4047243N	Crabtree camping area; head south along the spur trail, across the creek to a large number of sites ringing the meadow; food-storage box and toilet
12.19 🐾	203.5	17.3	11,110'	11S 379954E 4047528N	small tent sites on open sandy bench above creek; head south from trail
12.20 🐾	204.7	16.1	11,570'	11S 381322E 4047603N	3 tent spots under lodgepole pines between trail and creek
12.21 🐾	205.7	15.1	11,490'	11S 382326E 4048136N	head south to find sandy sites on the knob north of Guitar Lake and toward the west end of the lake; beautiful views to the Kaweahs and Mt. Whitney
12.22 🐾	205.8	15.0	11,500'	11S 382505E 4048032N	many exposed, sandy sites among slabs near the north shore of Guitar Lake; alpine scenery and beautiful views to Mt. Whitney; head south-west from the trail
12.23 🐾	206.5	14.3	11,910'	11S 382629E 4047999N	few small tent sites in sandy flats among slabs above Guitar Lake; head south from trail once east of Arctic Creek
12.24 🐾	206.6	14.2	11,920'	11S 383443E 4047422N	walk a short distance south to find sandy flats between many small tarns; uncertain late-season water

CAMP ID	N-S	S-N	ELEVATION	UTM COORDINATES (NAD 27)	DESCRIPTION
12.25 ⊗	208.2	12.6	13,280'	11S 384291E 4046766N	space for 1 tent on an exposed patch of sand with steep bluffs below; no water
12.26 ⊗	208.3	12.5	13,400'	11S 384334E 4046822N	room for 5 small tents in sandy spots among talus, mostly sheltered by rock walls; amazing views to the west; head east (upslope) from the trail on the last switchback below the Mt. Whitney trail junction; no water
12.27 ⊗	210.4	10.4	14,505'	11S 384473E 4048700N	Mt. Whitney summit; various sandy flats among boulders; views in all directions!; no water
13.01 ⊗	214.7	6.1	12,040'	11S 385616E 4046956N	Trail Camp; many sites in sandy flats among slabs, on both sides of trail
13.02 ⊗	214.8	6.0	11,990'	11S 385773E 4047005N	a few sandy sites among slabs at the far eastern end of Trail Camp
13.03 ⊗	215.6	5.2	11,430'	11S 386654E 4047420N	1–2 small sandy tent sites among slabs on open knob
13.04 ⊗	216.2	4.6	10,900'	11S 387116E 4047520N	small open sites on knob; excellent views but far from water
13.05 ⊗	216.3	4.5	10,840'	11S 387140E 4047638N	medium-size site beneath sparse tree cover; excellent views but far from water
13.06 ⊗	217.0	3.8	10,370'	11S 387445E 4047888N	Outpost Camp; very large area beneath scattered foxtail pines
13.07 ⊗	217.9	2.9	10,010'	11S 388197E 4048255N	little-used camping choices near the shores of Lone Pine Lake; head east along the spur trail for 0.2 mile to reach the lake

⊗ = no fires allowed
North-to-south distances are in miles from Happy Isles, while south-to-north distances are in miles from Whitney Portal.

RANGER STATIONS AND
EMERGENCY NUMBERS

	RANGER STATION LOCATIONS IN SEQUOIA AND KINGS CANYON NATIONAL PARKS	
Ranger Station (Distance from HI/WP)	**UTM coordinates where you leave JMT (NAD 27)**	**UTM Coordinates of ranger cabin (NAD 27)**
McClure Meadows (Section 7; 119.1/101.7)	11S 345299E 4116961N	11S 345381E 4116952N
How to get there 300 feet northeast of the trail, along the stretch of McClure Meadow with many campsites; easily missed when headed south.		
Le Conte Canyon (Section 8; 136.9/83.9)	11S 358394E 4106306N	11S 358333E 4106273N
How to get there Head 200 feet west on the spur trail at the Dusy Basin/Bishop Pass junction.		
Bench Lake*, ** (Section 9; 158.1/62.7)	11S 372078E 4091162N	11S 372101E 4091371N
How to get there Cross the outlet stream of the first lake south of the Bench Lake and Taboose Pass junctions. Then head northeast, for a total of 0.17 mile from the JMT.		
Rae Lakes (Section 10; 174.4/46.4)	11S 375133E 4074657N	11S 375198E 4074614N
How to get there Located toward the northern end of the middle of the three Rae Lakes. Head 250 feet southeast along the spur trail.		
Charlotte Lake (Section 11; 179.6/41.2)	11S 373686E 4070169N	11S 372820E 4070920N
How to get there From the JMT head 0.83 mile northwest on the trail to Charlotte Lake. The ranger cabin is just east of the trail, toward the northern end of the lake.		
Tyndall Creek* (Section 12; 194.4/26.4)	11S 375972E 4055618N	11S 375632E 4054817N
How to get there Head 0.58 mile southwest on the trail descending Tyndall Creek. The cabin is just west of the trail.		
Crabtree Meadow (Section 12; 202.9/17.9)	11S 379241E 4047246N	11S 379519E 4047234N
How to get there Head south across Crabtree Creek to the Crabtree camping area. Then walk 0.1 mile east along a spur trail to the cabin.		

* These stations are often unmanned due to budgetary limitations.

** The Bench Lake station is a canvas tent that is assembled when the station is staffed. The platform is not visible from the JMT when the cabin is down.

EMERGENCY NUMBERS		
Jurisdiction	**Trail sections**	**Phone numbers**
Yosemite NP	1–2	209-379-1992
Madera County Sheriff	4	559-675-7770
Devils Postpile NM	4	760-934-2289
Fresno County Sheriff	5–7	559-488-3111 (use when outside Kings Canyon NP)
Sequoia and Kings Canyon NP	7–12	559-565-3195 or 559-565-3341
Inyo County Sheriff	3, 13	760-878-0395 or 760-878-0235

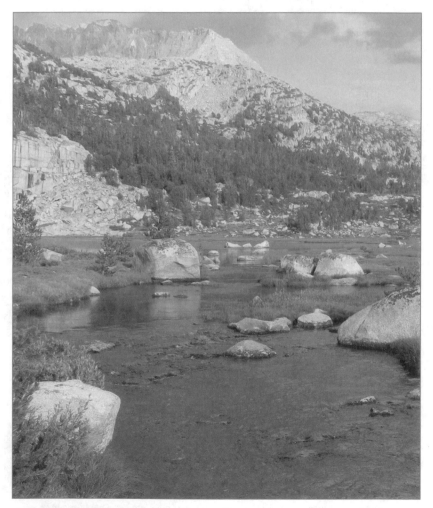

Lake just south of the Bench Lake junction

FOOD-STORAGE BOXES (BEAR BOXES)

LOCATION	ELEVATION	UTM COORDINATES (NAD27)
Little Yosemite Valley (Camp 1.01)	6,130'	11S 278409E 4179015N
Sunrise High Sierra Camp (Camp 1.17)	9,310'	11S 285790E 4185522N
south side of Woods Creek crossing (Camp 10.07)	8,530'	11S 371951E 4081607N
Arrowhead Lake (Camp 10.11)	10,300'	11S 374375E 4076443N
Lower Rae Lake (Camp 10.13)	10,560'	11S 374742E 4075037N
Middle Rae Lake (Camp 10.16)	10,560'	11S 375248E 4074161N
Charlotte Lake (Camp 11.02)	10,400'	11S 372816E 4070866N
Vidette Meadow (Camp 11.08)	9,550'	11S 374566E 4068867N
Upper Vidette Meadow (Camp 11.10)	9,945'	11S 375616E 4068176N
Center Basin junction (Camp 11.14)	10,500'	11S 377247E 4066060N
Tyndall Creek crossing (Camp 12.06)	10,965'	11S 376032E 4055967N
Tyndall Frog Ponds (Camp 12.08)	11,025'	11S 376215E 4055105N
Wallace Creek crossing (Camp 12.13)	10,400'	11S 377457E 4050483N
Crabtree Meadow (Camp 12.18)	10,700'	11S 379333E 4047146N

* The Charlotte Lake food-storage box and campsite are 0.8 mile off the JMT toward the northern end of Charlotte Lake.
**The food-storage boxes at Kearsarge Lakes have been locked; they were being abused as food-storage depots by JMT and PCT hikers.

Locations of food-storage boxes not on the JMT are available at **climber.org/data/bearboxes.html.**

JMT LATERAL TRAILS

There is much discussion about how to get to and from the Vermilion Valley Resort, generally known as VVR. This table clarifies the distances and elevation change required for the three routes between the Lake Edison junction and the Bear Creek junction.

WHICH WAY TO VERMILION VALLEY RESORT?				
ROUTE	TOTAL DISTANCE: QUAIL MDWS JCT » VVR » BEAR CREEK JCT	TOTAL ELEVATION: QUAIL MDWS JCT » VVR » BEAR CREEK JCT	ADVANTAGES	DISADVANTAGES
Edison ferry both directions and JMT over Bear Ridge to Bear Creek JCT	10.7 (3.0 off JMT + 6.7 on JMT)	+2,300, -1,200	• The entire length of the JMT • Beautiful view toward Selden Pass from the top of Bear Ridge • A well-graded, quiet, shady walk	• $19 RT for ferry • Ferry only runs twice a day (or +4.3 miles to walk one way)
Edison ferry and Bear Ridge Trail to JMT and JMT to Bear Creek JCT	8.5 (1.5 to ferry + 4.9 up Bear Ridge Trail + 2.1 on JMT)	+2,400, -1,300	• 2 miles shorter than other options • Much of the walk is shaded • Beautiful view toward Selden Pass from the top of Bear Ridge	• $12 for ferry + $10 for ride to TH • Ride to TH only twice a day (or add ~2 miles) • Not very scenic • +4.3 miles one way if ferry isn't running
Edison ferry and Bear Creek cutoff and Bear Creek Trail	10.8 (1.5 to ferry + 9.3 along the Bear Creek cutoff and Bear Creek trails)	+2,430, -1,330	• Truly beautiful walk • Follow a spectacular length of river for several miles	• $12 for ferry + $10 for ride to TH • Ride to TH only twice a day (or add ~2.5 miles) • Longest route—just barely • More of walk at lower, hotter elevations • +4.3 miles one way if ferry isn't running

TRAIL	TRAIL LENGTH	ELEVATION GAIN/LOSS	TRAILHEAD NAME AND UTM COORDINATES	TRAILHEAD ELEVATION	JMT JUNCTION	N-S	S-N	PERMITS	TOWNS ACCESSED
Panorama Trail (Glacier Point)*	5.5	+1,710', -530'	Glacier Point (11S 273226E 4178502N)	7,200'	Panorama Trail junction	2.8	218.0	Yosemite NP: Glacier Point to Little Yosemite Valley	Yosemite Valley, Glacier Point
Cathedral Lakes**	0.1	+0', -20'	Cathedral Lakes TH (11S 290501E 4194217N)	8,560'	trail to Cathedral Lakes Trailhead	20.6	200.2	Yosemite NP: Cathedral Lakes	Tuolumne Meadows
Lyell Canyon†	0.0	+5', -0'	Tuolumne wilderness permit office (11S 293760E 4194562N)	8,645'	Tuolumne Meadows permit station	23.1	197.7	Yosemite NP: Lyell Canyon	Tuolumne Meadows
Rush Creek	9.0	+500', -2,950'	Rush Creek TH (11S 312679E 4183712N)	7,235'	Rush Creek junction	39.9	180.9	Inyo NF: Rush Creek, Silver Lake	June Lake
Rush Creek	7.0	+600', -3,250'	Rush Creek TH (11S 312679E 4183712N)	7,235'	Thousand Island Lake junction	43.0	177.8	Inyo NF: Rush Creek, Silver Lake	June Lake
River Trail	6.4	+360', -1,750'	Agnew Meadows shuttle bus (11S 316610E 4172285N)	8,300'	Garnet Lake junction	45.4	175.4	Inyo NF: River Trail, Agnew Meadow	Mammoth Lakes
Shadow Creek	4.5	+360', -840'	Agnew Meadows shuttle bus (11S 316610E 4172285N)	8,300'	Shadow Lake junction	49.0	171.8	Inyo NF: Shadow Creek, Agnew Meadow	Mammoth Lakes
Devils Postpile	0.75 (N), 0.6 (S)	+135', -25' (N); +160', -25' (S)	Devils Postpile Ranger Station (11S 316127E 4166584N)	7,560'	northern (or southern) Devils Postpile junction	56.8 (57.5)	164.0 (163.3)	Inyo NF: JMT/PCT South Trailhead heading south; JMT/PCT North Trailhead heading north	Mammoth Lakes, Devils Postpile
Red's Meadow Resort to JMT†	0.3	+80', -0'	Red's Meadow Resort (11S 316934E 164899N)	7,710'	western (or eastern) Reds Meadow junction	59.2 (59.3)	161.6 (161.5)	Inyo NF: JMT/PCT South Trailhead heading south; JMT/PCT North Trailhead heading north	Mammoth Lakes, Red's Meadow Resort
Mammoth Pass from Crater Meadow	3.2	+710', -370'	Horseshoe Lake (11S 321674E 4164596N)	8,995'	lower Crater Meadow junction (Mammoth Pass)	62.0	158.8	Inyo NF: Red Cones, Mammoth Pass Trailhead	Mammoth Lakes
Duck Pass	5.6	+610', -1,670'	Coldwater CG/Duck Pass TH (11S 324448E 4162143N)	9,120'	Duck Pass junction	70.5	150.3	Inyo NF: Duck Lake Trailhead	Mammoth Lakes
McGee Pass	13.6	+2,780', -4,450'	McGee TH (11S 340819E 4157324N)	7,870'	Tully Hole (McGee Pass junction)	76.8	144.0	Inyo NF: McGee Creek Trailhead	Mammoth Lakes

TRAIL	TRAIL LENGTH	ELEVATION GAIN/LOSS	TRAILHEAD NAME AND UTM COORDINATES	TRAILHEAD ELEVATION	JMT JUNCTION	N-S	S-N	PERMITS	TOWNS ACCESSED
Fish Creek Trail and Iva Bell Hot Springs	18.4	+2,065', -3,710'	Red's Meadow Resort (11S 316934E 164899N)	9,200'	Cascade Valley (Fish Creek) junction	77.9	142.9	Inyo NF: Fish Creek Trail	Mammoth Lakes, Red's Meadow Resort
Goodale Pass	10.1	+690', -3,310'	Lake Edison TH (11S 322091E 4138859N)	7,825'	Goodale Pass junction	80.5	140.3	Sierra NF: Mono Creek Trail	Lake Thomas Edison, Vermilion Valley Resort (VVR)
Mono Pass	15.3	+4,200', -2,340'	Mosquito Flat/RockCreek (11S 345477E 4144341N)	10,220'	Mono Creek junction	86.6	134.2	Inyo NF: Mono Pass, Rock Creek	Mammoth Lakes, Bishop
Lake Edison†	1.5 (to ferry) 5.8 (to TH)	+550', -660' (TH)	Lake Edison TH (11S 322091E 4138859N)	7,825'	Lake Edison (Quail Meadows) junction	88.0	132.8	Sierra NF: Mono Creek Trail	Lake Thomas Edison, VVR
Bear Ridge	4.9	+100', -2,400'	Lake Edison road near dam (11S 324706E 4137456N)	7,735'	Bear Ridge junction	92.6	128.2	Sierra NF: Bear Ridge	Lake Thomas Edison, VVR
Bear Creek Cutoff	9.3	+1,030', -2,430'	Lake Edison road fairly near dam (11S 324269E 4136674N)	7,560'	Bear Creek junction	94.8	126.0	Sierra NF: Bear Diversion	Lake Thomas Edison, VVR
Bear Creek Diversion Dam	8.9	+400', -2,340'	Lake Edison road near Mono Meadows (11S 322527E 4134085N)	7,020'	Bear Creek junction	94.8	126.0	Sierra NF: Bear Diversion	Lake Thomas Edison, Mono Hot Springs, VVR
Florence Lake‡	4.2 (to ferry) 7.7 (to TH)	+250', -720' (to ferry); +630', -1,075' (to TH)	Florence Lake ferry wharf (11S 327911E 412421 8N), Florence Lake TH (11S 325027 4126806N)	7,330' (ferry), 7,350' (TH)	northern (or southern) Muir Trail Ranch cutoff	107.9 (109.7)	112.9 (111.1)	Sierra NF: Florence	Florence Lake, Muir Trail Ranch
Pine Creek Pass	17.8	+3,240', -4,000'	Pine Creek TH (11S 350320E 4136107N)	7,420'	Piute Creek junction	111.5	109.3	Inyo NF: Pine Creek Pass	Bishop
Piute Pass	17.1	+3,620', -2,410'	North Lake TH (11S 355703E 4121119N); North Lake parking (11S 356469E 4121476N)	9,260'	Piute Creek junction	111.5	109.3	Inyo NF: Piute Pass, North Lake	Bishop
Bishop Pass	12.0	+3,370', -2,295'	South Lake (11S 361066E 4114607N)	9,795'	Bishop Pass junction	136.9	83.9	Inyo NF: Bishop Pass	Bishop
Taboose Pass	9.6	+810', -6,160'	Taboose Pass TH (11S 381987E 409560N)	5,430'	Taboose Pass junction	157.8	63.0	Inyo NF: Taboose Pass	Big Pine, Independence

TRAIL	TRAIL LENGTH	ELEVATION GAIN/LOSS	TRAILHEAD NAME AND UTM COORDINATES	TRAILHEAD ELEVATION	JMT JUNCTION	N-S	S-N	PERMITS	TOWNS ACCESSED
Sawmill Pass	12.5	+1,200', -6,960'	Sawmill Pass TH (11S 385183E 4088677N)	4,595'	Sawmill Pass junction	164.8	56.0	Inyo NF: Sawmill Pass	Big Pine, Independence
Woods Creek	13.5	+110', -3,560'	Roads End, Cedar Grove (11S 358860E 4073060N)	5,036'	Woods Creek junction	167.7	53.1	SEKI: Woods Creek	Cedar Grove (Kings Canyon NP)
Baxter Pass	10.4	+2,190', -6,310'	Baxter Pass TH (11S 384385E 4078238N)	6,040'	Baxter Pass junction	172.4	48.4	Inyo NF: Baxter Pass	Independence
Kearsarge Pass (from north)†	7.4	+1,110', -2,560'	Onion Valley (11S 380384E 4070278N)	9,185'	Kearsarge Pass (or Charlotte Lake) junction	179.4 (179.6)	41.4 (41.2)	Inyo NF: Kearsarge Pass	Independence
Kearsarge Pass (from south)†	7.2	+1,345', -2,540'	Onion Valley (11S 380384E 4070278N)	9,185'	Bullfrog Lake junction	180.0	40.8	Inyo NF: Kearsarge Pass	Independence
Bubbs Creek	12.4	+0', -4,520'	Roads End, Cedar Grove (11S 358860E 4073060N)	5,036'	Bubbs Creek junction (Lower Vidette Meadow)	181.2	39.6	SEKI: Bubbs Creek	Cedar Grove (Kings Canyon NP)
Shepherd Pass	13.2	+1,755', -6,345'	Shepherd Pass TH (11S 385893E 4065164N)	6,300'	Shepherd Pass junction	194.3	26.5	Inyo NF: Shepherd Pass	Independence
New Army Pass, Cottonwood Lakes*	22.5	+4,080', -3,110'	Cottonwood Lakes TH (in Horseshoe Meadows) (11S 395230E 4034656N)	10,060'	Pacific Crest Trail junction west of Crabtree Meadows	202.1	18.7	Inyo NF: Cottonwood Lakes	Lone Pine
Cottonwood Pass*	20.4	+3,580', -2,750'	Cottonwood Pass TH (in Horseshoe Meadows) (11S 395165E 4034116N)	9,940'	Pacific Crest Trail junction west of Crabtree Meadows	202.1	18.7	Inyo NF: Cottonwood Pass	Lone Pine

* Alternative starting point

** This trailhead can only be used when traveling toward Yosemite Valley.

†Common resupply point

‡The trail lengths are measured from the trail junction between the two Muir Trail Ranch (MTR) cutoffs, a short distance east of the Muir Trail Ranch. This is 0.7 mile south of the northern MTR cutoff and 1.3 miles west of the southern MTR cutoff.

North-to-south distances are in miles from Happy Isles, while south-to-north distances are in miles from Whitney Portal.

Elevation gain/loss is calculated from the JMT to the trailhead.

Check out these other great titles from
Wilderness Press!

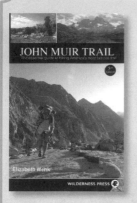

John Muir Trail

*The Essential Guide to Hiking
America's Most Famous Trail*

by Elizabeth Wenk   5½ x 8½, paperback
ISBN: 978-0-89997-736-2   296 pages
$18.95, 5th edition   maps, photographs, and
                                                   index

Elizabeth Wenk's authoritative guide describes the 220-mile John Muir Trail, running from Yosemite Valley to the summit of Mt. Whitney and onward to Whitney Portal. It provides all the necessary planning information, including up-to-date details on wilderness and permit regulations, food resupplies, trailhead amenities, and travel from nearby cities. Useful essentials are updated GPS coordinates and maps for prominent campsites (along with an updated list of sites along the trail), trail junctions, food-storage boxes, and other points of interest. The trail descriptions also include natural and human history—a must-have for any John Muir Trail enthusiast.

John Muir Trail

*Special Digital-Only Edition
for Northbound Hikers*

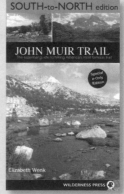

by Elizabeth Wenk   digital format
ISBN: 978-0-89997-772-0   maps and
$9.99   color photographs

This special digital-only edition provides all the necessary planning information to hike the John Muir Trail south to north, from Whitney Portal to Yosemite Valley.

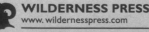
WILDERNESS PRESS
www.wildernesspress.com

... on the trail since 1967

ABOUT THE AUTHOR

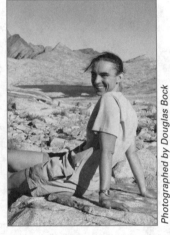

From childhood, **Elizabeth "Lizzy" Wenk** has hiked and climbed in the Sierra Nevada with her family. Since she started college, she has found excuses to spend every summer in the Sierra, with its beguiling landscape, abundant flowers, and near-perfect weather. One interest lies in biological research, and she worked first as a research assistant for others and then completed her own PhD thesis research on the effects of rock type on alpine plant distribution and physiology. However, much of the time, she hikes simply for leisure. Obsessively wanting to explore every bit of the Sierra, she has hiked thousands of on- and off-trail miles and climbed more than 600 peaks in the mountain range. Many of her wanderings are now directed to gather data for several Wilderness Press titles and to introduce her two young daughters to the wonders of the mountains. For them as well, the Sierra, and especially Yosemite, has become a favorite location. Although she will forever consider Bishop, California, home, Wenk is currently living in Sydney, Australia, with her husband, Douglas, and daughters, Eleanor and Sophia. There she is working as a research fellow at Macquarie University and enjoying Australia's exquisite eucalyptus forests, vegetated slot canyons, and wonderful birdlife—except during the Northern Hemisphere summer, which she continues to spend exploring the Sierra.